How'd You Do It??!!

How'd You Do It??!!

✦

Yes—weight loss is this easy

Angie Leszczak

iUniverse, Inc.

New York Lincoln Shanghai

How'd You Do It??!!
Yes—weight loss is this easy

iUniverse books may be ordered through booksellers or by contacting:

iUniverse
2021 Pine Lake Road, Suite 100
Lincoln, NE 68512
www.iuniverse.com
1-800-Authors (1-800-288-4677)

The information contained in this book is intended to provide helpful weight loss information for the general public. It is made available with the understanding that the author and publisher are not engaged in rendering medical, health, psychological, or any other kind of personal professional services in this book. The information should not be considered complete and does not cover all diseases, ailments, physical conditions, or their relationship to weight gain or weight loss. It should not be used in place of a call or visit to a medical, health, or other competent professional who should be consulted before starting any weight loss program, exercise program, adopting any of the suggestions in this book, or drawing inferences from it. Neither the author nor the publisher shall be liable or responsible for any loss or damage allegedly arising as a consequence of your use or application of any information or suggestions in this book.

ISBN-13: 978-0-595-41465-9 (pbk)
ISBN-13: 978-0-595-85814-9 (ebk)
ISBN-10: 0-595-41465-6 (pbk)
ISBN-10: 0-595-85814-7 (ebk)

Printed in the United States of America

Not that I have already obtained all this, or have already been made perfect, but I press on to take hold of that for which Christ Jesus took hold of me. Brothers, I do not consider myself yet to have taken hold of it. But one thing I do: Forgetting what is behind and straining toward what is ahead, I press on toward the goal to win the prize for which God has called me heavenward in Christ Jesus.

Philippians 3: 12-14 NIV Translation

"This book is full of truths that if followed, will lead to successful weight loss."

Dr. Christine M. Marcotte

I want to thank my husband who was faithful, loving, kind and quiet no matter what my size was. Above all I want to thank him for showing his excitement and happiness when the weight did come off. Without his continued praise and encouragement, this book would not be. I love you very much Glenn and you are my number one fan.

Contents

Introduction

"How'd you do it?"
"You must tell me EXACTLY what you are doing!"
"What diet are you on?"
"How'd you do it?"
"I know that—but *how* did you do it?"

I have repeatedly received these questions and statements from people who have known me through the years and have seen the lifestyle change I have made. I especially loved it when I had women I knew comment about how great I looked. One was the daughter of our friends who had known me since she was a little girl. We had taken her on a vacation with us many years earlier! When I went up to her and said hello, she stood there and did not say anything because she did not recognize me! She was shocked when I said who I was. She told me I looked great!

Of course, you have to love when people tell you that you look gorgeous, beautiful and fabulous. I eat it up! I earned it. Why should I not enjoy it? What is wrong with working so hard and reaping the compliments?

As I started thinking about writing this book, I wanted to have a little acronym for this book. Acronyms help people to remember big ideas in a little phrase or saying. I like them because you can write them on little pieces of paper and have a jump to your memory on whatever it is the acronym represents. The acronym I came up with rings so true in weight loss. I believe that without *one* of these parts you will fail.

BCD: Believe. Commit. Do.

Believe. What a powerful word. It means have faith or confidence in. In what will you have faith and confidence? You will have faith and confidence in yourself. I know this is a big problem with many you, but it is not the end of the line. You can believe in you. The more you believe in you the more you can gain in life. You are the only person who can change you. You need to believe in yourself that you can lose weight. Have faith in yourself. Believe you can succeed in anything you want. Believe that your body deserves it. You only get one body and the better you take care of it the better you will feel and the better all the parts will work together. (Would it not be awesome to lease a body the way you lease cars?) Believe in eating right. Believe that exercise is good for you. Believe that this is a lifestyle change, not just another diet or fad. Diets and fads are for a time. This technique is forever. It is a lifestyle change.

Commit. This word means pledge or bind to policy or course of action. Your course of action is to lose X amount of pounds. Your commitment is to make a plan and stick to it for the rest of your life. Make plans. Look ahead. Commit to yourself. Commit to having good health. Commit to making yourself keep your word for a lifestyle change and carry through on those changes which you have committed yourself to completing. Praise yourself when you do well and be hard on yourself when you cop out. A commitment means nothing if the heart is not in it.

Do. This word means perform, carry out, act, proceed, work at, satisfy, and attend to. Perform the eating rituals that will get you to your goal. Carry out the plans assigned to you by your nutritionist. The nutritionist told you what eating habits to change therefore you should do it. Work at it. We all will slip. Falling down does not count. Getting back up is what counts. Satisfy your need to feel good about yourself. Attend to your body. Do the exercises that you chose. Exercise on the days you have chosen. Exercise for the full amount of time you set for you. You will get no results if you do not continue with what you have put your mind to. Take care of your body. You only get one.

There are many reasons to lose weight. Medical reasons are always at the top of the list. Heart disease, diabetes, stroke, high blood pressure, hip problems, knee problems, respiratory problems, back problems and the list is endless. The second reason is to look good. Who does not want to look good? Some people lack motivation no matter what the need is for losing weight. It will take their doctor riding them and harping on them for them to start thinking about losing weight, and sometimes that is not even enough. Yet, with other people, it takes a life-threatening catastrophe like a heart attack, or at least the possibility of a disease coming to fruition soon for them to start thinking about lifestyle changes. Mine falls somewhere in the middle.

In April of 2004, my doctor told me I had elevated blood pressure. Who would not have elevated blood pressure with owning your own company, being a mom and an author? I did research on high blood pressure, because I did not want to have to take medication. I wanted to know what I could do to change that. I was concerned my sedentary lifestyle was as the root of the elevated blood pressure. I was right on the money. After confirming what I already knew, I decided I would begin to walk as a means to lower my blood pressure.

I had a unique workout schedule. It is a workout schedule that almost every American either has tried or is working on. Mine had the following rules:

1. I would walk when it was convenient

2. I would walk when it was not hot

3. I would walk when there was no rain

Then, those rules had to line up with the second set of rules. These were as follows:

1. Nothing that would make me sweat; just an easy walk to stay limber

2. Here and there; now and then; no concrete schedule

3. If there was time

4. If it was warm enough

5. If I did not have errands to do

Now one important note here is on the days I did not walk, I did not replace it with any other workout. There was no commitment. There was no reason to keep up the regiment. My blood pressure had started to go down. It was back in the normal range of 120/80. If I did not feel like walking, who was I to argue with my body and why should I keep my walking regular? Without a reason, there would be no commitment. Without a commitment, there would be no change. Without any change, there would be no results.

In May of 2004 one of my blood tests came back with a higher than normal blood sugar reading. This had been going on for the past two years and my doctor had not seemed too concerned so neither did I. She just said we needed to keep an eye on it.

In June of 2004 after continued "heightened sugar levels", I experienced some symptoms that scared me. I researched them on the internet, and the information indicated the possibility of Type II Diabetes. I knew people who had diabetes and saw how it affected their lives. I also knew my grandfather had it. I needed to have a definite diagnosis.

In late June of 2004, I called my doctor and requested a Glucose Tolerance test. I had the test done within a week and the results were not horrible, but I did not pass with great results either. I met with my doctor the following week to discuss my choices. I shared with her how I had done research on Type II diabetes and found out exercising and portion control, resulting in weight loss were the answers to getting my blood sugar back to normal levels. (I was not telling her anything she did not already know.) I further explained that I wanted the chance to make these changes. If I lost the weight and there was no improvement in my sugar levels, I would take the insulin as she prescribed. She agreed. My doctor gave me a referral to see a nutritionist. That is how it all began.

At this point, it would only be fair to address excuses for a lifestyle change. There is none. How is that? I have heard every excuse (I think in the world) and not one of them is good enough. But, to be fair, I have used them all myself. Being overweight is not an excuse, it is the reason you need to be exercising. Having no time is the most used excuse. Replace television with exercise. Experiencing fatigue ranks a close second on the list. Go to bed earlier. There is just no excuse not to exercise. It is a need, especially here in the United States where I would guess we rank high in sedentary lifestyles.

Now back to my story. I followed the instructions the nutritionist gave me. Without the nutritionist, I do not believe I would be at the weight goal I wanted to reach. (More details in the portion chapter.) What happened next was so important to my weight loss success. I then believed I could do it. I committed to a lifestyle change and I was going to do it. I took on the responsibility to make me better. I committed to walking every day, no matter what. I committed to portion control. I took on the responsibility of warding off Diabetes. This is what you have to do.

Never let anyone say you cannot do it. You can. It is mind over matter (or do you say mind over *body*?) There is also the matter of having self-control. Losing weight is achievable with a lifestyle change and if people continue to tell you it cannot, have those people call me! I was 180. I am now 131. With BCD (Believe, Commit and Do) it can be done.

Now that that is all said and done, let us get started so people can ask you *HOW'D YOU DO IT?*

1

What is the plan?

How many times have we heard?
"Eat five servings of veggies."
"Drink eight glasses of water."
"Exercise at least 30-45 minutes."
"You are what you eat."
"Increase fiber, decrease fat intake."

The list goes on indefinitely. If we know this stuff, because we have heard it so much, I have a question. Why do we not do it? I am just asking a question. If we can roll our eyes and take in a deep breath and then breathe out and say, "I know this" then why do our bodies look like we *don't* know it? I was just asking another question.

It is because we have head knowledge and not applicable experience. It is easier to hear and store, than hear and do. If we say we know it, and people do not see it (because of the unapplied knowledge), other people and us will think it does not work. But wait! It does work! I know it! I did it! I did it and it shows! I went from a women size 16 to a kid's size 16! You read that right. A kid's 16! The scale went from 180 pounds to 131 pounds! You can lose weight! I lost weight!

"I tried it and it didn't work." How many times and from how many different people have, you heard this statement? Weight loss is not a trying procedure. Weight loss and all the changes that go with that are a lifestyle change. A change that will last forever. It is a black and white issue. Eat right—lose weight. Exercise—lose weight. Obviously if we keep hearing the same stuff repeatedly, it would be worth trying it for a year or so. What could it hurt? It cannot hurt as much as not trying it at all.

I "tried" it because I had to. Diabetes II was on the edge of my horizon and there was no way it was going to make its full début. I knew making a lifestyle change was necessary. I had read it repeatedly. That was the only way I could live a healthy life. All the choices were mine. Change the lifestyle or suffer the consequences. As most of us are, we want the change and the result, without all the work that goes into the change to make the results happen. However, we do have to work at keeping our body in shape. It is not a given.

Something I heard much of when I started to explain long-term weight loss was "I KNOW THAT!" That is what we say. We *know* that! If we indeed *know* it then there is only one of two reasons for the weight not leaving.

- We do not know the meaning of the word know *or*
- We simply do not care

To define the word knows is as follows:

To perceive with certainty; to understand clearly; to be sure of or well informed about; to have perceived or learned; to have a firm mental grasp; to have securely in memory; to recognize by recollection, remembrance, representation or description.

To know is to do. I can hear you asking, "There is so much information out there, how can I remember it all?" Well that is true, but just remembering a handful of basics can expand your knowledge. Remember being in kindergarten and learning the ABC's? You could not learn to read or write until you had those imbedded in your head. This was because if you could identify the letters in the alphabet, you could put them together to form words, words to sentences and sentences to paragraphs. You could use them to your advantage. The same is true with weight loss and maintenance information.

What are the areas that we have heard so much about on nutritional information?

- Eating—what and how much
- Food—why do we need to eat the good and run from the bad
- Exercise—the calorie burner and why we have to
- Weight—what is it and where should it be

These are some of the common topics, which give us the keys to weight loss. Under each of these are at least a thousand subkeys that I could write on forever. However, the point of this book is to get you to understand how important each of the areas are and to apply it.

What is the reason you want to lose weight? The reason needs to be a real, long-term reason. None of this quickie "I need to lose x amount of pounds in a week for a family reunion." If that is what you are aiming for, this book is *not* going to work for you. If quickie weight loss is what you are looking for, just starve. Lose the weight, go to your family reunion and then continue what you were doing before the family reunion, which was overeating and minimum to no exercise.

What we are talking about here is a *lifestyle* change. This is *not* a fad. It is *not* a diet. It *is* a *lifestyle* change. This is *forever*! Now do not freak out on me. It is not as bad as it sounds. "Angie! Forever is a longtime." No. When you are diagnosed with a disease, forever is a longtime. Especially when it could have been prevented by some small, simple adjustments to your lifestyle. Forever is when you have to live with a disease for the rest of your life. That is forever.

Depending on your dietary needs, which we will talk about later, you may be able to eat anything you want! Yes. It is true! Ask me! Ask my husband! Ask everyone who sees me. I eat anything I want, in *controlled portions*. As I said, we will cover that later.

Right now, I want you to get a piece of paper. (I am waiting!). Now I want you to write down "Why do I want to lose weight?" Do not be shy about it. Put down <u>the</u> <u>reason</u>. Put down the truth. This is for you. This will be the sheet that tells you the why, when, where and how of this lifestyle change.

Write out every reason there is for you wanting to lose weight. Write out *exactly* what you want to accomplish.

- I want to look like a babe
- I want to feel better
- If it is a health reason:

  - I do not want to have a heart attack
  - I do not want to have a stroke
  - I do not want to have diabetes

My reason was that I did not want to have diabetes. I did not want to take insulin. But most of all, I did not want any of this because of something I had caused. If I had to take insulin it would be because of something I could not control, not because I ate too much, was lazy and did not want to be personally responsible for the mess I had made of myself.

You cannot believe, commit or do something for some reason that has no name. You cannot commit to an unknown. What is the reason? Why do you want to lose the extra weight? "Because my doctor won't shut up if I don't!" That is great! I love your doctor and I do not even know them! Doctors need to be active in their patient's road to successful weight loss.

My doctor was such an encouragement! I am glad she did not charge by the hour on my visits!

You need to know the exact reason, to the tee, so when you want to give up, you can look yourself in the mirror and say, "How bad do you want this? Is staying overweight worth not finding proper fitting clothes, having a stroke with partial or full paralysis, having a heart attack and not being able to be active? Is it worth not losing the weight?"

People now tell me I am gorgeous! I had a friend tell me I have always been beautiful but now I am "sculptured" beautiful. My friend says I now have defining features. No one told me that before. That was not why I wanted to lose weight, but it was a bonus! You need a tangible, *real* reason. So write it down and then let us continue.

At this point, in the book, you have probably either seen your doctor (If you have not, you need to) or have talked to a nutritionist and your weight loss now has a face. That face is a number. Let me say something here. It amazes me when people say, "I want to lose weight." Then when I ask how much they answer, "Oh I don't know." How can you commit to losing weight for an intangible number? How will you know you have reached your goal if you do not have a number? Some people say they will know by how they look. I suppose that could be true—but if you are like me, there are times I look or feel fat, and my weight says otherwise.

How can you make a change if you do not have a number? My doctor said I needed to lose five percent of my weight. That meant nothing to me. My scale does not measure in percents. Therefore, I went home and figured out what five percent of my weight was. That would have been about nine pounds. She had to be kidding me! How could nine pounds have me on the verge of diabetes? Most people would have taken the nine pounds, accepted it, and called it a victory. I was not accepting that. I am a finisher. I am an overachiever. I want to do it all and if I cannot do it all, I do not want it.

I researched the medical sites on the internet to find out what my ideal weight would be for my height. After researching on the American Heart Association, American Diabetes Association and several other reputable sites, the internet said 125-135 would be my ideal weight. I wanted to be 125. That was the best weight and that was what I wanted. That meant I had to lose 31% of my weight or 55 pounds. 31%! Yikes! (Five percent was not sounding too bad at that point.) My weight loss now had a face, and it was ugly.

Sometimes it is good to see what you have done to yourself. Is it embarrassing? Of course it is embarrassing! If you are anything like me, I want the best for me. I do not want a doctor telling me "if you had only lost the weight…" You and I are not going to hear this because we are going to make lifestyle changes.

Right here, at goal setting is the point where most people will give up because it is too hard. (If you do not believe me, look at the statistics of people who keep their New Year's Resolutions). Some people have already put down this book, wadded up their paper and put it behind them. Why have they crumbled up their papers? They have become frustrated because it is too hard, too demanding, too embarrassing. Nevertheless, you *MUST* set goals.

How can you have a plan without any goals? Goal setting is not as hard as reaching the goal. (For some people goal setting is a piece of cake.) But you must remember this chapter is talking about the specifics of the what, where, how and why of the weight loss. You cannot have one without the other.

As we work through the goal setting part of this, you must remember that a goal has to be realistic, as well as the methods set forth to accomplish your goal. Otherwise, you are setting yourself up for failure. Failure will occur within 30 days of a lifestyle change if you do not stick to it. The reason for failure is usually unattainable goals. To say you want to workout ten hours a day, seven days a week and lose 20 pounds a week is unrealistic. You will fail! This is a guarantee. You read it here! Moreover, if this is what you are thinking as a realistic method in reaching your goal, you did not listen to your doctor or your nutritionist.

Lifestyle changes are gradual because they need to stick. Your methods need to fit your lifestyle. That is why it is called a lifestyle change. You need to be able to reach and accomplish your weight loss goal, *no matter what*. That is how you will succeed. We have to make goals attainable. Now that does not mean there will not be roadblocks. (If you say you have never had a roadblock in life—you are a liar!) You may need to adjust the methods for a particular time in your life, due to circumstances. Remember roadblocks are unavoidable, but you cannot assist in setting up the roadblocks. Roadblocks are part of life, but they can be detoured. Let us move on.

On your piece of paper, underneath your reason for wanting to lose weight, you will now write three numbers across the next line on your sheet of paper. These numbers will be your road to weight loss success. These numbers will be the destination signs in your life. (Where you are, where you are going and are you going the right way?) The first number to write down is your current weight. "Angie, I don't want to write that number down!" Why don't you want to write it down? Is it embarrassing? Good. That proves you know you do not weigh what you are suppose to. Guilt and shame can be a good thing. My first number was 180. That is where I was. (Yes it is true. I was 180.)

Next to the first number, in the middle of the page, write the second number, this will indicate your targeted weight. (This is where you are going.) Now please be realistic about this. This is something my doctor pounded into my head every time she saw me. I explained to her, I would not become anorexic. If I were within a few pounds of my goal and stayed there forever *with what I was doing, which was my lifestyle change*, then I would be happy at that weight. My goal was 125. (At the writing of this book, I am at 131.)

The third number you are going to write down, on the far right side of your page, is the pounds that need to be lost. (This is the indicator telling you if you are going the right way). *Do not put this in percentage! Your scale does not read in percentage!* This number may shock you and seem unattainable and it could be if you are being unrealistic. However, if you talked with your doctor and your nutritionist, the number should be close to what you need to lose. My weight loss number was 55 pounds.

Now that we have those numbers written down, I want you to look at them and study them. Get them in your head. Burn them in your memory. Cry over them if need be. If you do not know what your goal is (where you are, where you are going and how far) how can you believe in something you know nothing about? How can you commit to an unknown? How can you do anything to attain something you have no idea what it is?

"I want to lose weight." This is a good start, but *"I want to lose 75 pounds"* is more convincing to me that you *do* want to lose weight. I now know which direction you are headed. The most important item is *you now know* where you are going! So get those numbers in your mind and remember them. There will be a test later.

Now that you know *why* you are losing weight, and how much weight you are going to lose, what are you going to do to lose the weight? What are you going to commit to and follow through on? These are the C and D of our acronym. The C and D contain two components. Eating and exercise. No one likes the word exercise, but it is an absolute in the success to your weight loss.

One of the most important rules of weight loss that you must burn into your thought pattern is that you have to reduce intake (food) and increase your output (exercise). It just does not work any other way. Unless you are under weight or already at your ideal weight, most people can afford to cut back on their portions. Again, it is a matter if you want to and how bad you want to lose the weight. Are you going to let food rule you? However, this section is not about food. It is about your plan what to do with the intake of the calories.

On the next line, you will write two numbers supplied to you by your doctor or nutritionist. These are calorie and carb intake. Depending on your dietary needs, you may need to use extra lines indicating fat, sodium or any other intakes your doctor wants you to monitor. Write these numbers under each day.

Look at all the numbers again. You have where you are, where you are going, the energy (calories) you have to spend, but how will you spend these? Let pictures of activities you enjoy or would like to do go through your head. What do you see yourself doing? Are you weight lifting, riding a bike, aerobics? The types of activities that have gone through your head are things you would enjoy doing. These are your means to exercise. Mine happen to be walking and aerobics. Write those ideas down on a separate piece of paper. If there is one, then write the one, if there are many items then write those down. This is now your plan of action.

So when will you exercise? This is the most important part, because remember this is a lifestyle change. Exercising is *not* an option. The words "I can't" are not a part of your vocabulary. Exercising is a need. You will need to make time for your exercise. Even on vacation time. So, on the next line write the days of the week across the page. Include Saturday and Sunday even if these are not going to be workout days. (You may have to swap days. That is life. At the writing of this book, my best friend had a car accident and was in ICU and I still worked out and was at the hospital almost every day).

You need to see the days you are committing to doing this. As humans, we are more prone to respond to what we see, in this case the days we are *required* to workout. It is important to know the exact components of certain measures to reach your goal. There should never be an instance of "I think I worked out..." You have to write it down, and see what it is you are doing and when.

Underneath the days, you have decided to workout, put the minutes to which you are going to commit to working out. Your doctor or nutritionist will have given you the time span that would be suitable for your workouts. Assigning minutes each day, and days each week is the usual regime. Mine started at 60 minutes, 5 days a week. I am now maintaining my weight and am walking 30-45 minutes a day, 2-3 times a week. You may break it up into two sessions, a day, if that works out for you. If you do, leave room on your sheets because we are going to write underneath the minutes.

As you are doing this, think about your life. When do you take the kids to school? When do you get off work? Do you usually go grocery shopping on Thursday's between five and six in the evening? These are all pieces of your life to think about when setting up your workout schedule. You need to consider every area of your life because this is a lifestyle change. You are going to be doing this for the *rest* of your natural life. Your exercise time needs to be sacred. In the exercise section, I will explain the need for the label sacred time.

As you look at the numbers that represent the time you are dedicating to working out, again let creative ideas saunter around in your head. Activities you can do to lose this weight in the periods you have written down. Add them to your previous list. Remember, "I can't" is not the right mindset. I believe you can do it. It is a matter of, do you want it bad enough to commit, and make the needed changes and adjustments to your life.

Here we are at the fun part. We know when we are doing "it". We know how long we are doing "it". How do we identify "*it*"? Go back to your extra sheet and look at the list of activities or exercise you wrote down. There could be one activity. There could be many types of activities. What you are going to do now is write down the activity or exercise you are going to do on the days you have scheduled a workout. This is as important as picking the time. It does not always have to be the same exercise everyday.

The dedicated workout time means nothing if you put down "lifting 300 pounds of weights" and you know you can't do this for more than five minutes, if at all. The "do" of this has to go with the "what". Go ahead and write down the exercise you have chosen for what day and let us move on because we will come back to this and cover it in more detail in the exercise chapter.

Your goal setting is almost complete. The last goal is the weight you will lose each week and month. According to the American Heart Association, a healthy weight loss is 1-2 pounds each week. An important note here is the less pounds you have to lose, the slower it will come off. So do not get discouraged. It will come off. Just continue with your lifestyle change habits.

Now that we have all the goals in place, the next obvious question is "*when will all the weight be gone?*" We all want the time of completion! "When will I look like a babe?" There is a definite equation that will put you within a few months of your goal. But remember this is dependent on your commitment and your body. *Note: not all bodies are the same!* They all react different.

My final goal time on my schedule was December of 2004 (the same year I started) because I was sure, my body would lose 2 pounds each week. Yeah right. Here I am and it is 2006 and I have lost all but six pounds. The completion time is a little beyond where I thought I would be weight wise and when. To be safe I would figure one pound each week. If you lose more you will be excited! On a calendar every Saturday, put the target weight. I have much insight to this and want to let you in on a secret. The weight does not always come off for your Saturday reading. *"You've got to be kidding me!"* No, it is true. It comes off when it wants. So do not get discouraged. It may show up Sunday, Monday, Tuesday or Wednesday! As long as the numbers are going down, you are going the right way.

You now have all of your goals in place. Congratulations! I now want to talk about the importance of all you have written down. Do you remember how long it took you to work out the details of your goals? Look at your sheet. It took time. It took time to go to the doctor. It took time to think about what you need to do. It took time to find out how you are going to reach your weight loss goal. It took brainpower. It took work. You now owe it to you to keep the goals.

The numbers and the exercise, if not applied, mean nothing and will do nothing. In addition, the weight will not stay off if you yo-yo your plan of action. Therefore, I have a solution for you. Because we are humans, we react better to rewards. In weight loss, you do not see the results for sometime, so there needs to be little rewards between the beginning and the end. Let me tell you how I did it.

I wanted to lose 55 pounds. That may not be a lot to you, but to me it was a mountain. My husband kept reminding me that it took me 15 years to put it on, so it will take some time to see it come off. Nah, nah, boo-boo! It took just over a year, with six pounds to go. So there you have it! Anyway, I knew to keep going, especially if it was going to take *years* I would need little bits of encouragement along the way. I made notes of the "rewards" I would receive beside my goals.

My first goal was 165. When I reached that weight, I had dropped down to a size 12. My clothes were hiding the weight I had lost, because I didn't have anything that fit properly. I made the reward four new pair of size 12 jeans. I was elated. It was what I needed to head for the next goal.

My next goal was 135 at which time I could buy a Coach purse. I did it! I went out and bought a Coach purse. It was great! I had reached my goal of 135 and there was my reward. I knew the reward was from me, but it still meant something. As humans, we respond well to the reward system no matter whom the reward is coming from!

My final goal is 125 and the reward is to be a new Jeep. I am currently at 131 and am looking eagerly towards the next goal. You must have a *noneatable* reward. A reward that you can see later and when you see it, you are reminded why you got it. You will have a sense of pride and accomplishment on seeing the item, knowing you can complete your weight loss goal.

Again, congratulations on finishing your plan of action. I know it was a lot of work. Believe me when I tell you it is worth it. We now need to put this all together so you can start on your road to weight loss success.

2

The Why of Portion Control

America is a wonderful country to live in. Unfortunately, we symbolize our prosperity as a nation by the quantity of food we consume. The problem is we are consuming extreme amounts of food. We eat much more than our bodies need. Our body was never designed to consume large amounts of food. We *make* our bodies consume large quantities of food. We then expect our body to work overtime to get rid of it all, and not make us look fat. Our body is designed to store the extra food as fat. Yet we get upset because we are overweight.

Let us look at this from another angle. You put ten gallons of lemonade in the gas tank of your car. The car does not run. Are you mad at the car? No. Because you know that is not how the manufacturer built it to perform. It needs gasoline. The same applies to your body. Food is your fuel. Thus, the food you put in needs to be the correct fuel so your body runs properly. If you do not give your body the required nutrients in the correct portions, it will use what you give it and put it where it thinks it needs it. Usually not where you want it.

Medical pictures have shown the human stomach to be roughly the size of an average sized woman's fist. If we could picture that every time we sat down to eat, we would have no obesity problems in our nation. Or at the very least cut down the amount of obese people.

Once again, freedom and prosperity have given us the idea that we need to "eat it all and lots of it." Thus, we are continually overfilling our tanks (stomachs). We continually stretch our stomachs beyond the normal capacity. If you eat a five-course meal, exactly how is that to fit in a stomach the size of a woman's fist? I am looking at my fist as I am typing this and there is just no way I can fit a five-course meal in my fist.

I have heard repeatedly you have to watch your portions. I did watch my portions. So I thought. Isn't that what we think? But what exactly is a portion? Many people say it is the serving on your plate. No. Everything has a limit. Everything has a function and a purpose, good or bad and that is what we are going to cover in this book. All the information you have heard probably a billion times about reducing portions, you are going to put it into action. You are going to make a lifestyle change.

When I went home after my visit with my nutritionist in June of 2004, I sat my husband down and told him what she had told me. I had to reduce my portions and probably reduce it by half. My husband looked at me in horror and said, "You have got to be kidding me! Does she want you to starve?" What my husband failed to realize was what a portion size was. None of us really knows a portion size, unless of course we practice the art of eating proper portions. Most of us think a portion size is what is on our plate, and in most cases it is not true.

During my visit with the nutritionist, she talked with me and asked me questions about my lifestyle. She had me list the exercise I did regularly. She asked about my eating style. What I ate. Where I ate and when I ate. She questioned me on my health statistics and after she took down these notes, she came up with a solution, a plan for my weight loss.

Before I continue, I want to make an important comment here that you need to read, write down and hang somewhere. When you follow up with your doctor or nutritionist, do not lie. Do not tell the nutritionist what they want to hear so you will look like the ideal patient. If you were properly eating and exercising, you would not be in their office in the first place, so tell them how it is.

Giving the correct facts is important because the nutritionist is going to base your dietary changes and needs on the information you supply. If you eat 75 Snickers a day and instead you lie and say, "I don't eat any snacks", the solution you are given will be wrong. The output of information is only as good as the original information.

The next area the nutritionist revisited was eating. She had me go through my eating habits. I started with the meats. I do not eat beef. I only eat chicken, fish and some pork. (If I were to talk to her today, my menu would only be chicken and fish. This information is important because if she felt I needed to cut down on red meats, she would see there was no consumption of red meat.)

I continued to tell her I was a major vegetable eater. (This was important because many of the good vitamins come from vegetables and fruits, so additional supplements were not needed.) Snacks were treats about three to five times a week. There was no soda intake. I only drank decaf teas with no sugar and decaf coffees with cream and sugar. (Once again, if I were to go to her today, I would tell her I no longer consume any dairy product because of allergic reactions. This would show her the low fat intake.)

I also told her, my husband and I ate out often because of our work schedules. But when we ate out, we ate at restaurants with real meals, not fast-food. I also pointed out that we traveled a lot personally, which lead to us eating out a lot.

The next item the nutritionist rehashed was my lifestyle. This is almost more important than the food section on honesty. If you paint a picture of an active lifestyle and your foods line up, the doctors may start looking at medical reasons instead of lifestyle reasons to your weight issues. The nutritionist asked me what exercise (s) I took part in, if any.

Unfortunately, doctors are so use to sedentary lifestyles, it is a surprise and a joy when they actually find a person who cares enough about their health to exercise and not become one with the television. I told her I currently walked about four or five miles each day and tried to do it every day, depending on the weather. (Upon the mention of Diabetes, my exercise increased because I knew that was one of the keys in warding off Diabetes II.) I told her that in the winters I did not walk, but watched my intake of food closer. I went on to tell her about my occupation and hobbies.

After I had told her everything she had requested, she smiled and said, "There's not much change needed. Portion size is the only area in which I suggest a change. Your diet needs to be this amount of grams of carbs and this amount of calories." (I am purposely not putting those numbers in because I want you to go see your nutritionist for your numbers, if you have not already done so.)

Remember we are all different and what I need is not, what you need. Please see your nutritionist or doctor so you know exactly what your dietary intake and output requirements are. I was a little frustrated on the portion size, as I thought about how much I ate and I believed I was within the portion control boundaries. Most of us think we eat healthy portions. Most of us are wrong.

After explaining my dietary requirements to me, the nutritionist went into much more detail on portion size. She showed me how to read packages. Specifically, how to read the calories, carbs and servings sizes. She gave me pages and pages of information showing me physical portion sizes, pages showing a particular food and the correct serving size with related carb count.

I knew nothing about carb counting nor how it affected me and thus I needed to be educated. One of the items she taught me was one carb = 15 grams. (Some people count each carb, but there is a shorter condensed version. She gave this equation to me.) When you read the package and see

30 grams of carbs, that equates two carbs. Be careful when you read the carbs, calories and fat. You need to look at the serving size first. What you see (the physical package) is not necessarily what you get to eat.

Now remember I thought I already ate nothing. My husband would not even take me to a buffet, because I only went up once! As the nutritionist went over the portions with me, I realized I ate two to three times the amount of food my body required! I was surprised because this information was only on the packages she had showed me so far! I had not even gotten into the sheets of items I ate daily.

I realized I was "overfilling" my tank. No wonder I looked like I was overweight! I was overweight! I was overweight because I ate too much food. (If portion control was a revelation to me—I am sure that two-thirds of Americans do not know their portion sizes.) How was it possible that I could be overeating when I thought I was under eating? How could I have thought I was eating healthy when in fact I was eating two to three times that which was required?

I was surprised one time when I was at the store and picked up a "personal" size frozen pizza. How many carbs could a personal pizza have? I cannot remember exactly what the carb count was, but I remember thinking it was awesome for having one pan pizza. Maybe this carb tracking was not going to be too bad. Then I looked at the serving size and the serving size was not the whole pizza. In fact, it was half of the pizza! This had to be a joke! The Nutritional Information listed on the package showed all the carbs, calories and such for half the pizza, not the whole pizza.

That is why it is so important to read the serving size *first*. First of all, this will keep you from consuming too much then feeling bad, and second, this will keep you from getting depressed when you realize how much you did consume in the past. Sometimes, the portion on the packages is fractioned down to less than half. Think about those luscious bakery muffins that are the size of a softball. The serving size the calories, carbs and other nutritional values are based on, is one fifth of the muffin! Then why do they make them so big?

Before I even continue, I want you to do something. Get a piece of clean paper. I want you to write the word *diet* in large letters. Now I want you to take that piece of paper and rip it up into little pieces. You have just seen your last diet. There are no more diets for you. This is indeed a life-style change. This is not going to be for the next month, the next year, or until I look good. This is forever. Now look at that little piece of paper lying crumpled up in the garbage and know you will never see another diet in your lifetime.

How many times have you been on your way to somewhere unaware of whoever had used your car before you did not put gas in it? Now you are looking at the gas gauge knowing there is not a gas station for miles. Hang on! You just went to the store and bought a case of pop! With joy beaming from your face you pull over, go to your trunk, get the case of pop and …
… why are you holding your breath? Are the thoughts going through your head something like "Do they know what they are going to do to that engine if they put pop in the gas tank?" Or "Are they stupid?!" I agree.

We do this daily to our bodies. It is so easy to go beyond portion control; we don't even know we are doing it most of the time. Here is one example we are all familiar with. We are on the road and hunger pains hit. We think nothing of swinging into a fast-food joint to grab a burger, fries, drink and oh! Do not forget to biggie it. The only item in that order that you are biggie-ing is your waistline. The burger and fries have only a small portion of nutrition. That nutritional statement in itself is a big if. If the burger is three ounces, if there are vegetables on it, if the condiments are minimal, if the bun is whole wheat and you eat about ten fries. So just taking a wild stab at that order, my vote would go for minimal nutritional value.

So why did you get it? We do it out of convenience. It is easier to whip through the drive-thru. Going to a sandwich place that you know has healthy sandwiches requires getting out of your car. Then, you have to pick your bread, veggies, condiments, and pick a side. Who has time for that? Well here is my rebuttal. Who has time to work off all of that fast food?

I will be the first to raise my hand, jump up and down and yell agreeing that it takes much time and energy to eat healthy. My time at the grocery store has increased by at least half an hour (if not more) to make sure the meals I am preparing are healthy. I now read the packages to see what the manufacturers are calling a "serving size" for this product. How many carbs are in any particular serving? Then I need to decide if I get this food item, is that within the allowance of carbs? I now officially hate grocery shopping. At least before becoming health conscience I could always run in to the store and grab "staples". Potatoes, pasta, cheese and hamburger are the staples of America. You can make anything from these ingredients AND the family is happy! Oh and you have to be on your guard for all the new low this and low that stuff. Often, you are better off just using the regular stuff and keeping within the portion size.

So why go through the hassle? To ruin your life is one idea. No. I am just kidding. I know this is going to come to a shock to you but hang in there with me. Get your phone handy just in case after reading this next statement you need to call 911 for medical help. *We eat to energize and to keep our body going.* Eating is not a hobby. It is not something to do when you are bored, angry, depressed or trying to get back at someone. Eating is fueling your body. It is just like your car.

Here in Illinois Ethanol is getting a push. It is about twenty cents cheaper than regular gasoline. What a deal! Except my owner manual does not list Ethanol as one of my fuel alternatives. In fact, it clearly states that if considering alternative fuel sources, please contact your car service department. Why would they say that? Ethanol was not one of the fuel sources available when they made my car. Now would it run on it? It prob-ably would. It is a gas substance. It probably would not run as well if I did not put in the fuel the manufacturer recommended. Good old 87 or 89-octane gasoline is what the manufacturer recommended, not Ethanol.

The same goes for our body. Yes, the body uses all the crud we put in it because it has no choice. Some energy source is better than no energy source, even though the quality is substandard. That is all it is getting so it is going to use it to the best of its ability. Except we know the body is not running at its best. It is not getting what the manufacturer recommended. Our recommended fuel source is veggies, fruits, fiber and water.

So how do you know what you need to eat? Vitamins are a good place to start. If you are how I use to be, the word vitamin congers up a bunch of letters that you know you need but do not know where they come from or what the need is. It is very interesting once you know what you need. What vitamins need what minerals and who looks to whom to do what. The body suddenly starts to look like a well ran factory, once all the parts get what they need.

You are the engineer and the maintenance person of your body. It will run according to what you put in and that means some parts may not work well, if at all. Let us look at some vitamins. Many of us know we need vitamins. What many of us do not know is how much and where are you suppose to get them. I am not going to go into a whole science class on vitamins and minerals. I just want to give you a hint of each vitamin. If you would like to read in depth about these vitamins and others, please get the book Staying Healthy with Nutrition by Dr. Elson Haas. It contains much more information on each vitamin.

I will keep my description down to the vitamin, the source, what it does for the body and how much you need. I think that much information will get you psyched enough to start paying attention to what you are eating. I am going to address fifteen vitamins. Many of these you will have heard of and may even know their roles. Some of the vitamins may even be new to you. So let us get started and see what it is that our body's need.

- Vitamin A: (beta-carotene) Vitamin A is found in leafy green vegetables (spinach, broccoli, mustard greens, Kale, lettuce). Vitamin A helps night vision, growth and healing of tissues, healthy skin, helps protect the body against toxins and lowers cancer risk. The Recommended Daily Allowance (RDA) is 5,000-6,000 for adult males and 4,000–5,000 for adult women.

- Vitamin B1: (thiamin) Vitamin B1, found in brans and germs such as wheat, rice husks, whole wheat, brown rice, oats, millet, spinach, cauliflower, most nuts, sunflower seeds, peas, peanuts, beans, avocado and pork. This vitamin has many bodily functions including but not limited to cellular production of energy, helps in the health of tissues and the nervous system, learning capacity in children, muscle tones of the stomach and helps prevent accumulation of fatty deposits in the arteries. The RDA is 1.2 mg per day.

- Vitamin B2: (Riboflavin) Many foods contain Vitamin B2 but not high amounts. Brewer's yeast, liver, tongue and other organ meats are a few in the meat group. Oily fish such as eel, mackerel, trout, nori seaweed, eggs, shellfish, millet, wild rice, dried peas, beans, dark leafy veggies are some of the other sources. B2 helps in cell respiration, maintaining good vision, healthy hair, skin, nails, and is necessary for normal cell growth. The RDA for an adult male is 1.6 mg and for an adult woman 1.2 mg.

- Vitamin B3: (Niacin) Vitamin B3, found in liver and other organ meats, poultry, fish and peanuts, yeast, dried beans and peas, wheat germ, whole grains, avocados, dates, figs, prunes, milk and eggs. Vitamin B3 stimulates circulation, reduces cholesterol levels in some people, and is important to healthy activity of the nervous system and normal brain function. Niacin has many functions including the health of skin, tongue and digestive tissues and synthesis of sex hormones (estrogen). The RDA for adult men is 18 mg. and 13 mg. for an adult woman.

- Vitamin B5: Vitamin B5, found in organ meats, brewer's yeast, egg yolks, fish, chicken, whole grain cereals, cheese, peanuts, dried beans, sweet potatoes, green peas, cauliflower and avocados. B5 supports adrenal glands to increase production of cortisone. It helps to counteract stress and enhance metabolism. The RDA is 10 mg. for adults.

- Vitamin B6: B6, found in organ meats, whole grains, fish, poultry, egg yolk, soybeans, dry beans, peanuts, walnuts, bananas, prunes, potatoes, cauliflower, cabbage and avocados. B6 helps in many clinical uses, but not limited to premenstrual symptoms such as water retention, acne, fatigue. It can also help with allergies, stress ulcers, depression, muscle fatigue, epilepsy, schizophrenia and kidney stones. The RDA is two mg. per 100 grams of protein.

- Vitamin B12: B12 found in most fish, crabs, oysters, egg yolk, milk products, yogurt, and tempeh. B12 is essential for metabolism, stimulates growth and increases appetite in children, increases energy and helps iron function better. The RDA is 3-4 mcg. This is per adult.

- Vitamin C: (Ascorbic Acid) Most citrus fruits contain Vitamin C. The fruits with the highest concentration are rose hips, acerola (yellow/golden) cherries, papayas, cantaloupes, oranges, lemons and grapefruit. Good veggies, which contain Vitamin C, are green peppers, broccoli, brussel sprouts, tomatoes and asparagus. Vitamin C, used in the formation and maintenance of collagen, helps heal wounds and maintains healthy blood vessels. The RDA for adults is 60 mg.

The following Vitamins B vitamins are known only by their chemical names.

- Folic Acid: Folic acid is a B vitamin. Folic acid found in green leafy vegetables. These include spinach, kale, beet greens, beets, chard, asparagus, and broccoli. Additional items are bean sprouts and wheat germ. Other sources are liver, kidney and brewer's yeast, oranges, cantaloupe, pineapple, banana, loganberries, boysenberries and strawberries. Folic acid helps to restore its own deficiencies caused by alcoholism, epileptics, psoriasis, stress or fatigue. The RDA is 400 mcg. in adults

- PABA: PABA found in liver, brewer's yeast, wheat germ, rice, eggs and molasses. PABA reduces aging of the skin. No RDA listed for PABA.

- Vitamin D: Vitamin D found in fish liver oil, egg yolks, butter and liver. Many products now come "fortified" with this vitamin. Vitamin D maintains healthy bones, prevents tooth decay and gum problems. The RDA is 10 mcg.

- Vitamin E: Vitamin E found in butter, egg yolk, milk fat, liver, vegetable oil, seed oil, or nut oil. Vitamin E is an antioxidant. The RDA for an adult male is 15-100 IU's and 12 -100 for an adult female.

- Vitamin F: (Omega -3 and Omega -6) this vitamin found in seeds, wheat germ, cod liver oil, soy oil, safflower oil, corn oil, and Linseed oil (flaxseed). Vitamin F needed for organ respiration, lubrication to the tissues and help reduce blood cholesterol. There is no RDA for Vitamin F.

- Vitamin K: Vitamin K found in dark leafy greens, alfalfa, kelp, blackstrap molasses, safflower oil, liver, milk, yogurt, egg yolks and fish liver oils. This is a very important vitamin because it is required for blood clotting. There is no RDA for vitamin K.

- Vitamin P: Vitamin P comes from citrus fruits such as lemons, grapefruits, oranges, rose hips, apricots, cherries, grapes, black currants, plums, blackberries, papayas, green pepper, broccoli and tomatoes. Vitamin P used for problems relating to blood clotting such as bleeding gums, easy bruising, bleeding ulcers, hemorrhoids, varicose veins, excess menstrual bleeding, nosebleeds, and the bleeding problems of diabetes. There is no RDA for vitamin P.

Whew! That was a lot of information. We are not through yet. Now that we know why we need to watch what we eat and what we are looking for, I want to give you some reminders on how to carry out this task.

As I have said several times, I was determined about avoiding diabetes and because of that, I stuck to the portion control as if the nutritionist were standing there at every meal I prepared. If I did not measure, measure, measure, it could cause me to have to take insulin for the rest of my life. Was food that important to me? Were having two more grapes worth it? Was that extra cookie with the two extra carbs? I ate because I needed to. I just ate too much. I measured and weighed everything to spec. Right down to the grape count. If my sheet said two-third cup, it was not a milliliter past that. If it said one-fifth muffin, I avoided it because I cannot cut straight. If the label said half cup, the liquid did not go *just over*, if anything, it was *just under* where it needed to be.

Now I say *did* because as the nutritionist had told me, after time you will be able to *see* how much you need. Your corneas will have portion sizes burned into them because you will have been doing it for such a long period. That is true. Although I am within a few pounds of my weight goal, portion control is a lifestyle. Now what happens when I hit 125? Are there no more portions? Even more so, because I reached 125 pounds because of portions, and to stay at 125 I will always need portion control. Would it have been easy to have "just a smidge" more? Who would have known? Who was going to tell my doctor? Me? Then what results would I have received? Not the ones I have today. You have to be devoted to you.

Without a commitment to yourself and to the weight you want to lose, you will continually slip back into the old ways. "What can one extra oyster cracker do?" "So what if I put five extra noodles in?" You have to be *obsessed* with portion control. You have to have a mind-set that you can kill yourself by overeating. It is a real fact. If your reason for weight loss is medical, you know what you are trying to avoid or fix. The key is you have to want it so bad that nothing can tempt you to "just this once". The extra food will give you extra weight, thus potentially giving you extra medical concerns. Whenever I am tempted to go *just over* I think of the insulin shots that could still happen if I were to slip into my old ways. If I eat as I use to, I will look like I use to look, thus in turn having any medical problems I use to have associated with the extra weight.

3

The How of Portion Control

So how did I do it? I was faithful to me. Again, no one was there with a checklist making sure my portions were to size. In fact, my son thought I was neurotic with the measuring. How else would I know what a portion was if I did not measure? Obviously, I did not know right offhand or I never would have had to go see a nutritionist. I did not change my son and husband's ways of eating, although after a time *my husband* adapted himself to portion control because he could see:

- He didn't need to eat that much to be satisfied and

- Portion control = weight loss

My husband did not, nor does he currently measure his food portions. However, a few eating habits he has learned from me.

- You do not need to fill your plate until you cannot see the plate anymore—and if you need to do this—use a small plate.

- You do not have to finish everything on your plate, and if you have extra, you probably did not measure correctly. If at a restaurant, you will have one to two meals to take home.

- Eating healthy does not mean you have to go without goodies. The goodies are in, but must be in correct portions and line up with calorie and carb count.

- You do not eat until you feel full. Feeling full is not a sign of satisfaction. It is a sign that you overate, which means you did not measure and had too much on your plate to begin with.

Yes it is that simple. Watch what you eat, watch the portions and the weight will come off. (My husband does not follow an exercise regime. His daily work offers him plenty of carb burning time.) Let me give you some different settings here so you have some examples of how to handle portion control in different situations. I have shared these repeatedly with the people who wanted to know "How'd you do it when…"

The holidays are big *not my fault* slip times. However, they do not need to be if you plan ahead of time. Here it is in the middle of summer and I am already planning for the holidays. Why plan so early? Because I know that I will have parties, dinners, goodie gifts etc. and people expect you to eat. By far, most holiday parties are buffets. They are cheap and you get lots of food. This is a warning! This is a warning! Stick to your dietary needs and portions no matter what! If you are unable to not fill every one of your food desires, maybe eat a much smaller lunch and then drink lots of water before you go to a party.

Not once in any of the diet books or lectures have, I ever seen or heard anyone say not to drink too much water. Water is our friend and it is good for you. It will save you in those times of weakness. Grab a glass or bottle of water and keep drinking until you come to your senses, which should be about the time your tummy is feeling full, with water. Let us continue with the buffet!

Here is a suggestion from a prior buffet connoisseur. Walk the buffet first. This way you can see what is at the five-mile marker of the buffet before you start to pile items on your plate. Obviously, you cannot put food back on the buffet once they are on your plate. Once the food is on your plate, unless it is something disgusting, you will decide to eat it instead of wasting it. Something else I have noticed. After you walk the buffet line, because of the different choices, you may not choose something because of another item. You may make a healthier choice simply by observing first.

This is *my* version of eating at a buffet. (Please note: I am specific in my descriptions here because I want you to see that I consider every arena of my health when I eat.) One of my dietary restrictions is (discovered after the nutritionist visit) my intolerance to dairy products. Therefore, I know from the start that anything with cheese or dairy is out of the picture. That is a no-brainer for me. However, if you like those cheesy little yummies think about the calorie and carb count. Have small portions. In my case, with no dairy, that takes about half of the buffet out.

I have now approached the meats. I do not eat beef, so it is down to any other meat that they may have, besides lunchmeat (run away from processed meats!). Turkey is a plus. Fish is good, and usually shrimp is on the buffet. Take note! Meat serving size is three ounce, each serving, six ounces for a daily intake. Depending on the meats, I know one ounce equals one carb. I now have to decide how I want to use the carbs my doctor assigned to me. Three ounces of turkey and three ounces of shrimp could use all my carbs, unless I did not use them all earlier on dips, crackers and condiments.

Therefore, if I want shrimp and ham rolls, I need to break it down to make sure the combination of *both* is nearly 6 ounces. I then need to include that to my carb count for the entire meal. Then tally carbs and calories for the day. If you go over 1/1000 of 6 ounces the portion police will not come out, but remember if you cheat, you pay. You cannot eat 20 ounces of meat as well as everything else and then gripe when the scale either does not move or goes up. You cannot have all the food you want and lose weight. It just will not happen. There are certain laws of nature written in cement, and that is one of them.

We are about a third of the way through the buffet. Veggies are also no-brainers. In most cases, you can have up to 3 and ½ cups of vegetables, nothing added, before you need to start accounting for carbs. I cannot even eat 3 ½ cups of veggies, not even in a vegetarian meal. What gets people in trouble is the blue cheese dressing for the celery, the ranch dressing for the cucumbers, the extra cheese and croutons for the salad and don't forget the extra side of dressing. *Everything* has a portion limit. (Most of these condiments mentioned should be consumed, in amounts no more than 1-2 teaspoons).

Watch the fruit. Fruit can increase your calorie count without much effort. Be careful. Although fruit is good for you, depending on the fruit you pick, you could blow your carb count out the window. This is why research on different foods is so important. Nutritional information is priceless. Remember, if you cheat you pay. (You will hear this many times throughout this book.)

I am at the buffet and I have gotten through the meats and the veggies. I have passed the delicious fruit selection and I am now in front of the casserole section. Every buffet that I have ever been to has one. I will take a teaspoon of what I think I might like. "What if you like something more than another?" Have a little more of one, and pass on the other. I do not eat breads, dairy or potatoes (because of the blood monitoring) so that takes out most of the casserole stuff.

I only have the desserts to conquer. Because my host went through so much trouble, I need to consume some of the deadly dessert. (Someone has to do it and it might as well be me!) If I have seen the dessert table before eating, I would "trade-off" for more dessert than main food items. If I wanted two pieces of cheesecake, I might only get three ounces of meat, or reduce how many casserole servings I take. On the other hand, I may decide to just skip the whole buffet and start at the desserts, thus guaranteeing me not eating anything healthy and blowing my carb and calorie count out the window.

Again, with your nutritionist's list of calorie, fat and carbs intake, you could adjust accordingly. I know (from experience) that standing in front of a buffet, or even reading a menu, trying to calculate carbs can become frustrating. But I assure you over time it will become a habit. You will look, calculate, and move on. I wouldn't do it if it didn't work. I'd have more key lime pie!

Also do not forget you can do trade off with your exercise. I do not recommend this unless you are committed to your exercise program. Once we consume our food, we forget the trade off the next day. We forget it in the next hour if we are honest with ourselves.

Eating is a mental game. That is how the mind works. Your eyes will only register what it sees and your mind quickly forgets all healthy ways of eating, when it is time to eat. I find having a friend can keep you from the eating whoas.

If you pick up a whole slice of cheesecake and split it with someone, your mind registers that you had "a piece of cheesecake". I do this a lot with my husband when we go out. We usually buy one meal and split it. Although I am physically eating half of a meal, the food on my plate was all eaten, thus my mind registers I ate everything on my plate. My tummy is happy, my waistline is ecstatic and I do not feel like a pig. Now maybe I am different, but it works for me. The same goes for any food, but I apply this to dessert when I am going to have it.

What about when we eat out at restaurants? Be meticulous when you eat out. Do not be embarrassed to ask or alter something that is on the menu! When I first started watching what I ate in portion size and selection, I was embarrassed to go to restaurants and ask for specifics. I would rather not go out. I did not want to "inconvenience" anyone. Huh? My husband always found this funny and would always ask, "Is this a free meal?" This question always perplexed me until I knew what he was asking. I was paying them to make my meal, therefore they should make it according to the way I wanted it. I mean it when I say that was a revelation to me.

I restrict my dairy intake to almost none. I now realize being an American, means everything comes with cheese. Sometimes cheese is not always listed, so if I am not sure, I ask. (Cheese is only second to ketchup.) One item that is like this is an omelet. There are places that put cheese in their omelets and some restaurants, which do not. I will not know unless I ask.

I also have realized Americans are big on potatoes of every size, shape and form. I do not eat potatoes that often. When I do, I eat them in teaspoons. Therefore, when I go to a restaurant I always opt for extra veggies instead of the potatoes. You should see the looks I get.

An absolute must is when dining out, you must watch your portion size. In restaurants, you usually get about three to four times the amount you should consume. Remember buyer beware! Ask for nutrition charts at restaurants. They have them so use them. Many restaurants now have special nutrition menus right inside the regular menus (Weight Watchers, Atkins and the nutritional info are already there for you.)

Limit restaurant eating to no more than once a week, if possible. Just while writing this book I got a call to go out of town. Dinner had to be on the road. I chose a sit down restaurant. My son wanted BBQ at this particular restaurant but as I went through their menu in my head there was not anything I could have. There was BBQ on a bun. There were french fries. There were no veggies, except coleslaw. My son said, "You can have salad." I did not want salad. I chose a Thai restaurant with chicken and veggies for my meal.

A valuable piece of information I got from the nutritionist was you can eat at restaurants (preferably not fast food—but you can if you wish), just half the portions. (Sometimes, thirding to fourthing is needed.) I order whatever I want and ask for a to-go container right away, unless there are other people with me with whom I can split the meal. When my food comes I half it and again the body registers that "you finished your plate". Occasionally, I order a kids meal. The portions are perfect, you do not have to half it, and your body thinks you pigged out because you cleaned your plate! It is all in your mind on how your brain registers food consumption. If you do not see the extra food, you do not want it, thus you do not eat it.

On another night I went to another one of our favorite BBQ hangouts (which does offer grilled veggies) and ordered my normal dinner. I asked for a to-go container right away. When the food arrived, I took half of the meal and bagged it for my husband for his lunch the next day. When he went to eat it for lunch he could not believe what I had brought him was *half* the meal. He thought I had not eaten anything and brought him a whole meal!

The other dining areas that are tricky, but are not restaurants, are coffee shops. There are many hidden calories and carbs at these places, so be aware and prepared. That does not mean you cannot have a cup of coffee. With my particular dietary needs, because of the dairy intake limits, I thought I could not have coffee because I could not have any dairy related products. Thank God for nondairy creamer. When I go into a coffee shop just for regular old jo and they don't have nondairy creamer, no order. I regulate what goes in my body and if I cannot find what I am looking for then there are no substitutions. I have to deal with the effects. Therefore, I am fussy. Also, be careful with cakes, cookies and other delicious yummies when selecting your coffee.

Family schedules and jobs can make it difficult to eat right, but there are ways to get around this. If money is tight and eating at home is the only choice, look into Crock Pot cooking. I love this way of cooking because you throw everything into the pot in the morning and when it is time to eat you only need to get the plates. Chicken cooks up wonderfully in the Crock Pot and you can throw all your veggies in there and away you go. What is also convenient about this way of cooking is you can make a ton of food and then once you eat, break the remaining food down into individual serving containers. This way when you are running out the door, just grab a container out of the freezer for lunch. When it's time to eat your lunch, all you have to do is warm it up and you have stayed within (depending on what you put in the container) your calories and carbs, and still had a satisfying meal.

How do you handle the annual office party? The rules to this are similar to the buffet, but because most office parties are not buffets, this has some different rules. First, do not stand around the table to talk. For whatever reason talking and eating go together, and usually we are not paying much attention to the quantity we are consuming.

I had heard once that from Thanksgiving to New Years Day people on the average, consume 500 more calories a day than at other times in the year. This amount included alcohol as well. If you drink, you should look into the calorie and carb count on your favorite drink. I do not drink thus I do not know the exact calorie count on alcoholic drinks. I have heard from people that those calories can add up to 3,500 a week and 15,000 extra calories in 30 days! However, do your research.

Still yet, another arena of eating that could be disastrous to your life-style change is recreational eating. What does that mean? I am not talking about snacking. (I'll talk about that in a few minutes.) Recreational eating is eating just to be eating. There is no hunger, no reason, and no value. If you do recreational eating, it will take you beyond your calorie and carb daily intake. This is a guarantee. If you are hungry and it's not mealtime, drink water. This will usually resolve the issue of feeling hungry.

Here is a big, big, big revelation that everyone needs to realize and understand. If you are craving a candy bar, have a miniature candy bar, or a portion of a larger one, and satisfy the craving for the candy bar. Otherwise, what is going to happen is you are setting yourself up for disaster. You are going to eat ten baby carrots, seven low fat crackers, and a half bag of microwave fat-free popcorn. You are still going to want the candy, and you will end up eating it too! Remember you also ate everything else. You are going to be in trouble calorie and carb-wise. Just satisfy the food craving in the allocated amount. If a candy bar is two carbs and you have two carbs you can spare, go for it, but also make sure you are within your calorie count.

How do desserts fit into this new lifestyle change? What if you are a dessert person? Some people eat dessert because of culture or tradition. Some people eat dessert simply because of habit. Now what are you to do? You can have them. I never said you could not. Depending on your nutritional needs, your doctor or nutritionist may have advised you otherwise, but I did not say you could not have them. I said portion, portion and more portion control.

Most people (including me) have a hard time portioning desserts. They are yummy and we want to eat them until we burst. I would rather forgo dessert than have to portion. But, I have my weaknesses too. I am that way with key lime pie. I would eat it until I turned green! If you have to have dessert watch the portion size, be meticulous on the measuring and choose your dessert carefully. Maybe opt for sorbet instead of ice cream. Fruit pie instead of the custard pie. Choose oatmeal raisin cookies instead of the double chocolate.

Let us take moment and deal with if *you* are to bring something somewhere. We have talked about going to some place and eating what they have prepared, but what if you have to bring something. I had a girlfriend who had to bring a dish to pass at an office party. She called confused because she did not want to seem like the health fanatic. (I advised her to go for it!) But she knew the dish she brought, would probably be the only one she would be able to eat and stay within the limits her doctor set for her. I advised her not to worry about it. She could bring whatever she wanted. She told me she wanted to bring a vegetable tray and I told her most people do not gripe about veggie trays. They are healthy and you can snack on them all-day long with little to no guilt. She took the veggie tray.

Do not be ashamed to be health conscious. You would be amazed at the number of people who are influenced by the way I eat. All they have done was seen me choose my food and eat it. I did not get to lecture them on the benefits of why I eat the way I do. I didn't even get the chance to tell them why they should change their eating habits!

One of the easier pits to fall into, in weight loss is "the snack". (Snacks are not to be confused with recreational eating. Snacks are eaten because you are hungry and between meals.) Here you are between meals and the tummy monster makes his appearance. You have to eat something! Do not satisfy your hunger with empty calories. I am just as guilty for "just grabbing a little something", as the next person is. If you are policing your diet, there is no such thing as safe "just grabbing something" unless you have your own snacks on your person or in your car. Because of my lifestyle change, I now carry trail mix, or a healthy, nonperishable snack in my car as well as a case of water. (Remember I was allocated snack carbs—keep the snack within the numbers.) If you want to take or make your snacks on a daily basis, keep the snack in proportion with your carb and calorie count and choose wisely.

I love salads, but they are not a grab and go snack. An alternative to this though is a veggie drink. I also have yet to find a turkey burger on whole wheat bread in a three-ounce form at any fast-food restaurant. (Do I hear an idea for a franchise business? I am just kidding Glenn!) Chicken is always available, but not on wheat and you cannot eat chicken on the run without a bun. Yes, there are chicken nuggets, but they are usually in heavy breading and usually, dry, so you usually need to soak them in some form of condiment. It is hard to find something that will satisfy me, but also will be good for me. What a task! Start looking at food with the attitude of "what can you do for me". It is up to me to have the perfect snack to hold me over.

I know some people have to have snacks because of the medication they are taking. This is not a problem. Just make sure your snack is healthy. Peanut butter and apples are tasty and nutritious. Trail mix is a plus and you do not have to eat much to feel fulfilled. Just choose wisely. Besides, once you start to look good and feel better, you do not want to "go the other way," and undo all the hard work you have done.

Think about all those vitamins we talked about awhile back. Guess where the best place is to get most of them? Veggies! Always, always, always opt for veggies. Choose for snacks, main dishes, whenever and wherever. The only trap with veggies is the accessories. Butter, cream sauces, dips, dressings. You can have them. I have them. The servings of the condiments need to be in minuscule amounts. When I ask these veggie yummy accessories "what can you do for me", they smile and say "Nothing. But I sure taste good don't I?" The accessories have no nutritional values. None, nada, zip, zero. They contain no other nutritional values other than calories. On the carb scale, these condiments count as zeros, usually. On the calorie side, let us not talk about it.

Particularity is the key to the food part of your life. I have researched different cultural eating habits and the best ones are the Eastern diets, specifically Mediterranean. Why are these best? Because they use the good oils, especially olive oil. They keep their meats to a minimal. When they do have meat, they choose good meats. Fish and poultry are the main choices. Almost no beef and again if they have it, they keep it as lean as possible.

When you look at your plate here in America, meat takes up half, if not more space on the plate and a few veggies. We have it the opposite of what it should look like. Veggies are our friends. Veggies are our life source. We can do without meat, but there will be much trouble in our bodies without our veggies. Have you ever heard of a meatitarian? Our plates should be mostly veggies and small to minimal amounts of meats and the meats are to be of minimal fat content. Fish is the best with poultry close behind.

It will take some work to get use to your new lifestyle of eating, but it is worth it. People will be upset with you and embarrassed when you order or prepare food. Who cares what other people think. When those numbers start diving on the scale you will start looking at cookies, cakes, ice cream and all that "good" stuff as your enemy. Food is your energy source and just like your car, you want to put in the best to get the maximum results.

Portions are of the utmost importance. Oh, the horrible eight letter word. Buy measuring cups, spoons, scale, and USE THEM! These will become your best friends. Buy "fun" colorful ones. There are some cute ones out there. They even have scales that talk to you. Do not take a second mortgage to get these items because you will not need these forever. Eventually you will be able to "eyeball" the serving size. Using these measuring tools daily will help you succeed in your portion control. But remember to use them for what they are.

One cup is one cup. Not one cup with "a little extra" thrown in". Do not measure a teaspoon with "an extra shake". Of course, I'll tell you again, there are no portion cops, but if you are going to cheat, you need to realize you will pay. If you cheat, you have forfeited the opportunity of griping because your scale is not moving or is moving up. The almighty portion needs to be that which it is, a portion. Therefore, when you buy a whole chicken, you get to eat "a portion". You do not get to eat the whole chicken.

Exactly what is a portion; a serving of food on your plate or bowl? Sure. That is the picture we have in our heads. However, is it in the right picture? We need to reprogram our thinking about portion sizes. I have found some items that are common to the normal American household that can be a help, especially when measuring tools are not available. See Appendix D.

This should be a start for you, but there are books that list thousands of items in portion sizes. Believe me, once you start losing the weight and you are already measuring, you will know by sight, what the portion needs to be. It is wonderful to know what to eat, but now we need to know how much to eat. According to the American Diabetes Association Exchange List, we should be consuming these serving sizes, most of which count for one carb: (more portions in the back of the book)

- Bagel, 4 oz..............1/4 bagel (I ate half and thought I was doing great!)

- Bread, 1 oz..............1 slice (this means ½ sandwiches, not full!)

- Pasta (cooked)..........1/3 cup (no more endless bowls of pasta!)

- Oyster crackers.........24 (yes Virginia, you need to count them out.)

- Pretzels....................3/4 oz. (most packages tell you how many pretzels)

- Baked Beans.............1/3 cup (yes, you need to measure)

- Corn.......................1/2 cup (this is a starchy vegetable, so we have to measure)

- Stuffing....................1/3 cup (so much for Thanksgiving….)

- Muffin, 5 oz.............1/5 (1 oz.) (How many of us eat the whole muffin?)

- Fruit cocktail............1/2 cup (includes the juice)

- Grapes....................14 small grapes (most bunches have more than that)

Do you now see how easy it was for me to overeat and yet think I was not? How many of us take the bag of oyster crackers with our can of chicken noodle soup (which with one can of water added, is four servings) and just keep adding crackers until the soup is gone? How many of us pick up a healthy nut and fruit muffin for breakfast and think you are doing your body good? When the truth is you ate five times the amount you were suppose to. (Even with bran, there are no exceptions to the ingredients.)

Take a moment and think about grapes. Usually you grab a bunch or two because that is what the grape commercials say. "They are good for you" is what they tell you, but what they forgot to mention was the serving size is 14 grapes, not fourteen bunches of grapes. So let us take a quick look at a "healthy" breakfast.

You grab a bran muffin and two bunches of grapes and do not forget the large coffee with cream and sugar to wash it all down with. Right there you just ate probably close to ten times the amount you should have consumed for breakfast. Do you see how easy that was to over consume? Yet it did not feel like it. It did not look like it. It was all healthy ingredients! You were not even stuffed after that continental type breakfast. That is why we have to read and measure. Again, the American Diabetes Association lists these as the correct serving sizes we should be consuming:

- 6 oz drink=1 serving = ¾ cup
- Muffin = 1.5 oz = size of an egg
- French fries = 10 (obviously no biggie-ing)
- Fruit = 1 med pc or ½ c. chopped or cooked
- Veggies = 1 cup raw leafy greens or ½ cup cooked
- Breads and grains = 1 slice or ½ c cooked grains
- Dairy foods = 2 cups milk or yogurt, 1.5 oz natural cheese (i.e.: cheddar), 2 oz processed cheese (i.e.: American)
- Cookie = .5 oz (yes that's a point before the 5, and most deli cookies weigh 4 oz)
- Candy corn = 22 pcs. (Yes, you need to count them out)

- Whoppers = 18 pcs.

How can I not have to carry around measuring cups and spoons? Below are a few visuals provided by Wichita State University that will help when measuring tools are not available. There are more listed in the back of the book.

- 1 piece of fruit or potato = the size of a light bulb
- ½ cup = the size of a racquetball
- 3 oz meat = deck of cards or cassette tape
- 1 tsp peanut butter = one dice

Reading food labels will now need to be a way of life. Is it a pain? Yes. Do you look like a health freak reading labels? Yes. Does this make you depressed and wonder why you even bother eating? Yes. Does this help you cut down on your portions so you can lose weight? Yes. But, that is what I did. There is nothing in this book I didn't do myself.

Remember as Americans we already eat too much. Although, I heard on the radio one morning the Australians are heavier. The announcer said there is a problem with the Australians breaking their toilet seats! I am not kidding! To make matters worse, here is the not so funny part. The manufacturers of toilets are making heavier toilet seats instead of encouraging people to lose weight. Amazing.

Almost every person in America could cut down half of what they eat and still be fine. Most people could almost third their portions and still be fine. That is straight from the nutritionist! Think about the way you prepare meals. Are you preparing meals in large quantities? I always wanted to make sure I had enough food in case someone dropped in unexpectanty. In all the years I have been married do you know how many people dropped in for dinner? Not one single person has dropped in for dinner. Do you know who ate all that food for those people who I thought would drop in for dinner? That is right. We did. But, guess who gained the weight. We did.

We are what we eat. If we eat, too much we will weigh too much. This opens the door for other health problems besides overweight. Remember Diabetes II was peeking over my horizon. Then you have the knee problems associated with being overweight, and the hips. The list is endless.

What I am about to say will go against all grains of saving if you are on a budget, but believe me it's for your own good unless of course you have a will of steel. Buy snack size and DO NOT save money! Save your waistline! The extra .25 cents is not worth the extra 25 days of trying to get the extra pounds off.

I am so impressed with how the snack industry is making it easier to be able to have their products. I do not know how you are, but I would rather do without instead of going through the torture. The torture of getting the Oreo bag and having to take out three, while the other fifteen cookies sit there and look at me with their beady cream fillings. I would rather buy the snack bags and know I can consume the whole bag. There is much mind game playing in this alone.

What happens when you have the three Oreos? If you are at all like me, you know there are fifteen more cookies and you start running calculations through your head like ticker tape. The calculations fly trying to figure out if you can afford to have one more in comparison with what you have already consumed and may consume throughout the rest of the day. Too much work. That is too much brainpower for another one or two cookies. But if you have that little snack bag—which is usually the same carb or calorie count as your regular serving size, your body celebrates the victory of being able to eat a WHOLE bag. A whole bag of anything! You ate it all! You can go without feeling guilty for the rest of the day or dreading the scale in the morning. It is well worth the extra 25 cents.

Another tool to help in the eating and weight loss of your lifestyle change is The Glycemic Index. Although it has always been, the Glycemic Index has come to the forefront of the weight loss industry. It became familiar to me when I was trying to keep my blood sugar low and although I had cut my portions to almost nothing, my readings were still high. I did a search on the web for high sugar levels and this is when I learned of the Glycemic Index. It is the best information I have yet received in my lifestyle change.

Although fruits are good for you, if you are diabetic or need to control your sugar level to keep from having to take insulin, fruits can in fact bring you more harm than good. (I have experienced this myself.) According to many internet sites I have visited on the Glycemic Index, any food over the 50-index level breaks down fast. The higher the number, the faster the breakdown rate, which will keep your blood sugar elevated.

So what is this Glycemic Index? According to The American Diabetes Association, the glycemic index ranks carbohydrate foods based on how they affect the body's blood glucose levels. Again how fast or slow the particular food is broken down, thus how fast it is absorbed. There is much more information on this in books focused on this topic or visit The American Diabetes Association web site.

An area in your life style change, that could become a pothole in progress (and should be patched immediately), is meal planning. I hate it. Believe me if I lived by myself, soup, veggies and nut bread would be all you would find in my kitchen. I do not like to be creative when I cook. I do not like to think a lot about preparing meals. I would rather go out all the time and deal with the hassle of picking from the menu at a restaurant. But my family likes variety. So I had to sit down and develop a new list of staples that would be good for me and yet satisfying and pleasurable for my family.

If you do not plan your meals, you will grab a meal on the road and when you pickup one of these meals, you usually are not thinking about the nutritional facts of whatever the food is you are grabbing. If you find yourself in that predicament a lot, make a binder with the restaurants that you frequent, and highlight the items you have decided are the healthy choices. You can go one step further and just put several meals together from that particular restaurant and when you pull in, grab your notebook (that you have in your car) and read off the list. This is a no-brainer. It will take a little bit to put it together, but once you do, it is a snap for dinner.

Many restaurants now have low carb and calorie menus. As I mentioned before an option is to pick up their menu, highlight the items you would order and when you go there all you have to do is pick from the highlighted items. Planning is the key to not overeating and not overeating the wrong foods when you are just "grabbing something" for dinner. Although the convenience of grabbing a meal was worth it the night before, you will not be thinking about the convenience aspect when you get on the scale in the morning. Been there, done that.

Do not skimp on carbs! Is that not the opposite of what is being sold to the public today? An important statement we know, but cringe at because we know the cost of carbs is this statement, don't skimp on carbs. We need carbs for fuel and we forget this. Yes with fewer carbs, you will lose weight faster, but you will be tired. You will not want to think about working out, not to mention not having the energy to exercise. Once you realize you need carbs and add them back in (usually in large quantities) the weight will return. So eat properly from the beginning. Lose the weight at a slow pace and it will not return.

I have passed my two-year anniversary of keeping the weight off. I still have a few pounds I want to lose, that my doctor says I cannot lose because of my age. However, I have kept the weight off for two years with no yo-yoing. It was a gradual loss and it stayed off.

Is it worth the counting? Yes. Will you feel better? Yes. Will you miss any of if? No. Does this need to be forever? Yes. Watch your portions and watch your waistline dwindle away.

4

Tracking Your Weight

To look and feel good, you have to work at it. How many times have you heard this saying and could picture yourself choking the person speaking this? *"I am working at this and the dumb scale is broken!"* Um…excuse me, over here. Here I am with my hand up. Yes. Sorry to agitate you, anymore than you already are, but the scale is, uh, how can I say this and not offend you? The scale is saying what it feels. It is telling the truth. I know from experience. That one hurt, but scales do not lie, unless of course you have many clothes on—which I hate when the doctor's offices do that. Get over it.

Did you ever meet a scale that you loved or even slightly liked? Here is the subject that you probably thought I would never address, or at least was hoping I would forget about. However, how can you talk about weight loss if you do not have a scale to show your success or lack of success? The scale is the key tool to weight loss that everyone hates—until it shows the number desired. Your scale is your tool to success. There is no way around it. You need to become best friends with your scale. How else will you be able to measure your success?

The number on your scale, when you stand stark naked on it, with both feet fully on the scale, is what you are. Accept it. Swallow your pride. To be truthful with you, are you not a little proud of how much you have gained? No? Good. You put it on and now you have to take it off. I know it stinks. I know where you are coming from. The scale only shows what is on it. I have been there and done that. I swore I was still 140 when I was 180. No one could believe I was 180, but I was. Thank God for little favors, but now when I show the before and after pictures, no one can believe it was me. It feels good and guess what else has happened? I now like getting my picture taken now and I like my scale. What do you know?

If you are avoiding the scale, you already know there is a problem. How do I know that? Remember, I have been there. I no longer growl at my scale. In addition, when I eat more than I should, I do not get mad at the scale. I was the one who decided to eat after 8 o'clock (one of the big weight loss secrets) and to have a few cookies when I was fresh out of carbs and calories. I knew it and I had to pay. (See even I am not flawless.) The scale showed it with the extra one, two pounds. Was it worth it? No. However, I knew that before I began to eat. All of us know it. We just choose not to follow the rules.

The answer to the all-knowing, lying scale, which always shows a higher weight than you are, is to buy one of the new digital ones. This will solve many problems. First you will not be taking off x amount of pounds because you were not sure where that darn line stopped. The line is never where it should be. Even if you get the first line on the zero, when you get off the scale, it is one or two lines on either side of the zero. Buy a new scale.

There are scales on the market that do everything for you, except measure out your portions! (I am sure those are not too far in the future!) Seriously, buy a digital scale. You do not have to calibrate it. You will not have to make sure you are standing at the exact angle to make sure the line is exactly on the zero. What you need to do is go and buy a digital scale and weigh yourself the day before you go to the doctor (or an hour before, if feasible) and "sync" your weight with their scale. Their scale is right (unless it is one of those old iron weighted adjustable ones and has not been metered out).

When my digital scale weighs me and shows the magic number (whatever that may be), there are no questions. That is who I am. Am I happy?

Sometimes I am. Sometimes I am not. I am especially happy when the number decreases, but it will not increase if I have not given it the opportunity to do so.

Of course, you could count on how your clothes fit, and some people do, but if you are aiming for a particular weight, there is no way around getting on the scale. Now honest to God and you can call my husband about this, I hated my first scale I owned and I knew that I knew my scale was broken or it was a liar and hated me! Then, to add insult to injury, the doctor's scale *always* weighed me in 10-15 pounds heavier than I was! (I always thought I wore ten pounds of clothes to my doctor appointments.) Please! Get real! Get over it!

Unless your scale is as old as your grandmother is, the scale is usually within 1-2 pounds of your actual weight (clothed or naked) if not exactly what you weigh. I understand this is a hard idea to swallow, but I have been there, tried to justify the weight and failed. The scale was right and I was just living in a fantasy world.

Once you are honest with yourself (which can hurt and usually does) and once you make your dietary changes the numbers will go down. If you watch your portions and you exercise, they have to go down. Do you remember I mentioned the laws of nature? This is one of them. The only reasons the numbers will not go down are if you are cheating or you have already reached your desired weight. So you only have to face the "bad" weigh-in once (get on the scale, see the real number—the real you). Everything else is downhill from there.

I have found many people do not know how to weigh. I can hear you scratching your head. You get on the scale, look down and that is it. No, that is not all there is to weighing. A few parts play an important role in weighing yourself accurately. The time of day you weigh is a big one. I know people look at me and give me a face as if I am from another planet, but listen to what I am saying. Follow me here.

I get up at 6:30 in the morning. I eat at 7:00. I eat again at 12 and finish the day with dinner between 5 and 7, and try my best at finishing dinner before 8 p.m. (I will discuss this time issue later.) Now here is the question. When do you think I weigh the least? I will give you a moment. Time is up! What is your answer is? That is right! The best time to weigh is when you first get up! So why would I weigh myself at 12 o'clock one day, 10 o'clock another day, or 2 o'clock any other day? I will never have a consistent reading or path to track my weight. It is impossible. Consistency is one of the keys in tracking your successful weight loss.

When you weigh in it should be on an empty stomach. Hence the word empty. There is nothing in your tummy and that equates less weight. Thus, when you get up in the morning after a good night's sleep that is when you should weigh. Now if you ate after 8 p.m. the reading is going to be off. This is because of the fact there is a high chance your dinner (or late night snack) was not fully digested. Thus, there is extra food still sloshing around in your stomach. (Usually 1-2 pounds) Besides, it is not good on your stomach eating that late anyway. Remember when you get up in the morning you weigh yourself, making a note if you indeed ate after 8 p.m. However, there is one more item before your weigh in.

Here is another question. You have just slept 7-8 recommended REM peaceful hours. (Yes Virginia this is possible.) No interruptions during the night and you feel great. What do you need to do before you get on that scale? Remember you have been sleeping for eight hours. Can you guess what that is? Tick tock tick tock. Time is up! Yes! Once again, you have gotten the answer right! Go to the bathroom!

However, here is another key to tracking your weight. All elements need to be the same on every day. Weigh yourself naked. I freak out when I go to the doctors office during the day. I have clothes on and I have probably eaten at least one meal. They are not weighing me for what I am.

Therefore, after they weigh me, I have them write down the weight *I took* that morning so the doctor has an accurate reading.

I am a fanatic about my weight and it took me almost losing my temper with a nurse to get them to start writing down the weight I took at 6:30 in the morning. I worked hard to lose this weight and I want my chart to reflect the truth! Otherwise, it looks like my weigh is fluctuating like the temperatures in Chicago! One hundred thirty, one hundred thirty six, one hundred forty, one hundred thirty three, one hundred thirty five. But the nurses never make note of what time I came in, how much clothes I had on, and how many meals I had eaten, unless I ask them to.

Obviously if I go to the doctors at two in the afternoon, I am going to weight three to five pounds more than the morning weight. I have two meals in my stomach and I am fully dressed and if it is winter, make those five to seven pounds for the sweaters and boots! In addition, I have probably not gone to the bathroom!

Time to weigh is important. Preferably, early in the morning, but that does not always work for people. If you are like my son, he is not a morning person. He sleeps until the last second possible, so he can roll out of bed, into his clothes and off to wherever life is leading him.

To recap. It is important to weigh in at the same time everyday. That way if you weigh in at two p.m. everyday, everything is going to be the same. Even with two meals in your tummy! And last, but not least naked is the best way to weigh yourself. But if you are self-conscious, weighing with the least amount of clothing is better and be sure it is as close to the same type and amount of clothing every time you weigh. Do not weigh in one day with just your nylon undies on and the next morning it is too cold so you weigh in with your flannel nightgown and booties on. You are going to show 1-3 more pounds than the previous day weigh in.

You are now ready to get on the scale. You have gone to the bathroom. You are now emptier than ever and naked as a jaybird. What is the magic number? You write that down and now make a note of what time you weighed yourself. If this time is a good time (the weight may not be a good one but you still need to write it down because it will get smaller) then that is the time when you should weigh everyday. It does not need to be on the seconds but I would try to do it within an hour on either side.

Do not be afraid of the daily weigh in. I have heard so much controversy over this issue. Do not weigh daily, weigh weekly, weigh monthly. I suppose there is no right answer unless you want the right weight answer. Here is another problem for you to solve. Let's say you weigh in the first of the month and then weigh once or twice throughout the month. Then next month's weigh in says you have gained six pounds, do you know how long that is going to take you to get off? Probably another month, if not longer and you will not know what caused the gain, unless you are journaling or watching what you eat.

I weigh in every morning. That way if I am one to two pounds heavier I can get that off in about one to two days. In addition, if the weight is higher, I know what caused it. I am almost right on the money every morning with my weight. I know what I ate and what stays on longer. Pizza and Chinese are heartbreaks. One to two pounds and it takes about two days to get off. It is not worth it to me. Therefore, I know that if my family wants Chinese, whatever the previous meal is, needs to be smaller than normal, or eat tiny, tiny Chinese portions. 1/32 of an egg roll, 1/8 teaspoon of rice, 1/8 teaspoon of chop suey, no I am just kidding…. However, sometimes it is sneaky and it will not show up for one day. Sneaky sneaky Chinese food.

I tell everyone who asks me how often they should weigh, I tell him or her to weigh in daily. Once you bite the first number and realize you are in trouble, it is downhill from there. That is if you are committed. Remember that cheating shows. Maybe not directly to your waistline, but on the scale it will show every time.

If you binge and go on a cheesecake meal for two days, or an ice-cream marathon, do not look at the numbers on your scale for a week or a month! It is going to be bad news. There is no question about it. On the other hand, if you are watching everything you are eating you will lose weight. If you are exercising how you are suppose to you will lose weight. Or if you have hit your targeted weight, the weight will stay the same. If you are still on the road to losing, one pound a week will be what the scale is taking off. It is that simple.

Your scale only reflects what you are putting in and using. The equation is simple. You consume the fuel (reflected in calories and carbs) and that needs to be equivalent if not less than the energy you will use. Thus, your weight will stay the same if you have reached your goal, or you will lose weight.

I know people who hate exercise and do everything and anything to avoid it. (I do not hate it—I just do not like to know I am doing it.) People would not have a weight problem if they decreased their intake of food, a lot. People are surprised when the scale number keeps increasing. You have to spend the energy you have deposited. You will keep the weight if you do not use it, and it then shows as a "deposit" on the scale. Just like your savings.

If you keep putting money in the bank and do not spend it, the balance goes up. If you keep depositing and are turning around and spending it, the balance goes down. Do you see how easy this is? I have an analogy for everything! Reward is the result of spending in this area in life! Spend away!

Weighing is the report card to whether you are doing what you are supposed to be doing. There is no other way to know exactly how much you weigh, for the good or the bad. Let us consider your clothes that are getting too big. That reflects inches lost, but I have gone down a size and my weight has not change. I continued my lifestyle change and then the numbers on the scale went down again. There is no right or wrong answer to how often to weigh (daily, weekly, and monthly) it is just how much correction you want to do. I would rather correct one or two pounds instead of four to eight.

Consider other indicators of weight loss. There is the almighty BMI. This is an acronym for Body Mass Index. This number is the identifier of whether you are obese or not. What does this BMI mean? Body mass index is a measure of body fat based on height and weight that applies to both adult men and women. There are many BMI calculators available on the internet. However if you would like to figure it out yourself, here is the equation and scale provided by the National Heart, Lung, and Blood Institute (NHLBI) as a part of the National Institutes of Health and the U.S. Department of Health and Human Services. Calculating body mass is as follows:

Weight/(Height in inches) x (Height in inches) x703

For example, a person who weighs 135 pounds and 5 feet 5 inches tall has a BMI of 22.5. This is what that number means:

Below 18.5 = Underweight
18.5 - 24.9 = Normal
25.0 - 29.9 = Overweight
30.0 and above = Obese

It is just one more measurement to help keep your weight in line. If that is not enough incentive here is something else for you to think about before you take your scale and wing it out the window. A survey done by the weight loss website, sparkpeople.com revealed:

Thirty five percent of people name the bathroom scale as their number one source of weight loss motivation, beating out compliments, the mirror and increased energy.

I would guess the reason behind that would be there is no way for the scale to lie. It says what it feels and there is no way for it to get around that.

"I want to lose twenty pounds this month! Help me!" Losing 1-2 pounds a week is reasonable. I know there are those "diets" that guarantee you to lose 25 pounds in a month. That is not safe. The rapid weight loss is not good for your body and most of all it is not going to stay off. If I am going to lose the weight, I do not want it showing up anytime soon, if ever again.

If you are consistent with your lifestyle change, you should be losing one to two pounds a week, consistently. Now let me let you in on another little secret. The closer you get to your goal, the slower it comes off. Those last six pounds I need to lose, do not want to leave for nothing! I suppose these are the original six, that started this whole weight gain and they feel they have squatter rights or something. What they do not realize is that they have to leave.

If I am eating my x amount of carbs and x amount calories and I am spending them with my exercise routine, bye-bye six pounds and it wasn't fun having you here either! Please remember that it took time to gain all the weight you put on. You did not just wake up one day and have fifty extra pounds on you. It may have felt like that, but that is not how it happened. So losing the weight will take time too. Maybe not as soon as you like, maybe longer. That will be up to you on how committed you are to your lifestyle change. Commitment equates change. Cheating equates no change, or very little. It is your decision.

I am a writer and I like to write in every area of my life, and that goes for my weight loss as well. When I first started losing weight, I kept a journal. I wanted to *see* what was happening. I knew I was losing weight, but I wanted to be able to go back six weeks and see where I was when.

In my case, I typed up a monitoring sheet. You can put it in a little journal book, scribble on scratch paper or whatever and however you want to do it, but you need to write it down. On my sheet, I had several labeled columns: (see sample of journal in Appendix C.)

- Complete Date—this is more relevant to woman because that "time of the month" adds water weight. (So don't freak out—it accounts for about two pounds, but will disappear after "that time".) Also, I put complete date because depending on your goal this may extend over several years so you may not know which April you were looking at.

- Time—in case you could not be consistent and weighted in at a different time.

- Weight—actual—not wishful thinking (phony numbers won't get you anywhere and could make you depressed if not psychotic). Remember this is not up for public display. This is simply a record of where you were, where you are going and how far you have to go.

- Blood pressure—I was monitoring this, it is good to know, and it is amazing to see the numbers go down once the weight starts coming off—two for one!

- Blood sugar—I was also monitoring this, with an added column for time, because I was monitoring at different times each day. Again this is not bad to know even if you go to your doctor quarterly to have this done.

- Exercise—amount and type (mine was walking listed in time and miles). This is important in overseeing your weight. If the weight has been at a plateau for three months, something is not right and you will need to look between your eating and your exercise. How will you remember three months from now what you did? This is important especially if you are mixing up your exercise routines. You may find that when you walk, it does not give you the results as fast as lifting weights. There is never too much information.

- Notes—this can be whatever you want but I used it so I could put in what I ate that day or maybe something, that would reflect weight gain. (Chinese food adds 2 temporary pounds that don't leave for a few days, must be the MSG!) I also found that if I ate fruit and a small dessert my blood sugar was high. I knew this because I could go back and look and when these two were present in the same meal, so were the high sugar levels.

Many people like the idea of writing information down. They can *see* the progression or sometimes the lack of progression. I had one woman I was consulting about her weight loss progress. She could not understand why the weight was not coming off. To see where problems were occurring, I suggested to her to keep a journal and that way in the next week or so we could go over it. She would not do it.

Some people do not like to write their habits down because it then makes them accountable for their failure. I say this with the deepest respect, because I do not know one person who if they are doing what they are supposed to be, does not want to see the results! Who would not want to brag, grab their sheets and say, "Look, this is how I did it!" Only those who are not watching their portions or not exercising do not want to see the negative results!

Writing down the good or bad in your journal needs to happen, especially in the beginning. Why do you need to write everything down? Adjusting your lifestyle will be a daily ritual. I had problems with my blood sugar for several weeks. I could not get it to go down. I poured over my sheets and could not find anything that appeared to be contributing to this. (This was disheartening, as I believed my exercise and changes to my eating behavior would change my sugar levels.) To make a long story short, after much research it was my instant oatmeal in the morning that was throwing my numbers off. I kid you not.

I researched the Glycemic Index and because of the processing method of instant oatmeal, it breaks down fast. I had to change to the cooking type oatmeal. I would not have known that had I not been journaling my progress. In my case I wanted (and still want), to know what my weight was each day and I wanted to know what I ate, and how it was affecting me.

As humans, we would rather not eat something if we have to write it down. If you eat, no matter what it is, write it down. If you ate a whole package of Oreos, you need to write it down. I would encourage you to put a note in the notes section about what drove you to do it. There is always a reason. I say this seriously because if you can see that you are eating in large quantities because of stress, you need to note this. You will need to watch and keep an eye on your eating habits when those times arise.

If you cheat, you pay. No matter what the reason is. Your body does not care if you are upset or can justify why you ate half of a cheesecake. It does not care. Your body works a certain way and that is how it is.

In most cases, as silly as it sounds, we will not have three cookies if we have to write it down. Instead, we will have one, because we do not want to have to write the extra two. Although no one but you and possibly your doctor would see your food journal, it is another one of those mental games.

Let me say something here though, the journal is only as good as the information in it. If you are fudging the weight numbers so it appears you are losing one to two pounds a week, you are going to be in trouble. If you are putting in the recommended portions instead of actual portions, in a month you are not going to know one true weight from the next. Then when you go to the doctor's office, you will know you lied. If you cheat, you pay.

Remember doctors are not stupid. If you say you did everything right down to the last measurement, and you have not loss any weight, your doctor will know. These are just laws of nature. Have you ever seen a person with the flu gain weight? No. Why didn't they gain weight? Because food makes them nauseated, they are throwing up, thus, they do not eat, and in turn, they lose weight.

To have a successful weight loss trek you need to make sure you know your weight at any given time. When I get on the scale now in the morning, I almost to the tee know what I will weigh. It does surprise me on the loss, not because I do not think I will lose it, I just do not know when it is going to show up. This is so important because as I said earlier I have planned on the weight showing up on Saturday mornings. You will never guess what happens. It is usually not there. So I realize it will come off, I just need to stay on the path. That is my job and that is your job. Apply what you know and the weight will come off. It is that simple.

Let me go over the most important action to monitoring your weight one more time. Weigh, weigh, weigh. Remember, if you do not weigh everyday, how will you know how to adjust to stay on course? Again I have to say I have heard many people's reasons of why and why not to weigh yourself daily. As I mentioned before, I have decided that people who do not want to weigh everyday know darn well, why they are not weighing everyday. I have names and numbers to prove it.

Maybe you could give your scale a hug now and then, just to let it know you love it and let it know you realize it is only reflecting your actions. I know that was a tough one to read. It is the truth though. The sooner we realize we are the cause of our weight gain and that aliens do not come in during the night and pump us with high calorie foods, the better off we will be.

Let us talk about plateaus while we are in this chapter. Plateaus. I hate plateaus. Does anyone love plateaus? Raise your hands. I see no hands. Plateaus are another one of those potholes of weight loss. Remember plateaus mean something. Yes, I know it is hard to believe, but remember I know what I am saying because I have been there at 180, done that at 130ish.

I remember when I hit 167. I was so excited because I had a reward coming at 165. Do you know I plateaued for a month and a half? Now how did I know that? My chart I kept told me every time I had to write it. Plateaus are crossroads in the journey of weight loss. When you hit a plateau, you know it. You know it because the number does not change. 167, 167, 167,167,167. Day 14, 167. Day 30, 167. Day 45, 165. What was that? Get off and back on the scale. 165. Hooray! Plateau over.

There is much patience needed when a plateau happens because if you are sticking to your lifestyle change, the weight has to come off. If it is not coming off, you are either cheating or at a plateau. I know of several people who once they hit a plateau and were there for a while, and remember they had lost weight, in large amounts; they then went back to their old ways! I have meditated on this and to this day have not grasped this. If you lose 50 pounds and you plateau there for a month and let us say you are stuck there forever, what have you loss? You have loss 50 pounds! So why go back to the old way?

So how do you survive a plateau and find the strength and gumption to continue? When I hit the 167-pound plateau, I had an important decision to make. Day one to five on a plateau is survivable. Six and beyond you need to start talking to yourself and convincing yourself to stay on the straight and narrow road.

I am at 131. I want to be at 125. I had come to the realization when I was at 134, since I had been there for over four months, I could stay the weight I was, because of my age. Then one day I got on the scale and boom! 131! Have I changed anything? No. If I continue my eating and exercise regiment and this is not my weight, it will come off. If I am this weight a year from now, chances are this is my weight. There are many forty-something's that would like to be my weight.

As I tell everyone I talk to about this, if you are doing what you are suppose to be doing, the weight has to come off. Unless of course you have reached your goal and if you have, you wouldn't be reading my book. If you have reached a plateau, DO NOT GIVE UP! Keep going! What is the worse that can happen if the plateau weight is where you "land"? You are now x amount of pounds lighter than you were x amount of months or days ago.

Stay put. Stay on the path. If your goal is to lose 100 pounds and you and your doctor have decided on that weight goal and you plateau out at 50 pounds lost, stay on track! I have lost 50 pounds! Why would I give it all up, if I were unable to lose the last six? I look good, I feel good, my blood sugar, cholesterol, blood pressure and BMI are perfect, what else can I ask for? Remember this is a *lifestyle change*. You have to keep going. You have decided to believe in yourself that you can do it, you have committed to doing it, now do it!

5

Exercise—Workout—Just Love IT—Whatever IT is

There are many facts in life that people tell us repeatedly not to do. Do not drink, do not overeat, do not drive too fast, do not swear, do not make hasty decisions, do not overspend do not do not do not. The exception being, I have never heard anyone so far, and I am now 42 years old, say "don't exercise" and I know many people.

I do not know about you but my mother never told me "don't go out and play!" My gym teacher never told me "Take it easy, you are doing too many sit-ups!" My track coach never told me "slow it down you're running too fast" and my latest marathon coach never told me "Ang! Slow it down! You are walking excessively fast! It's not good for you!" Do you see where I am going with this? There is nothing wrong with exercise. Only good comes out of exercising. Better circulation, better energy levels, better thinking abilities and the list goes on.

On the other side of the list, I have heard 1000 to one, the excuses for not exercising. (Most people will not call them excuses, but that is what they are.…excuses.) Here are just a few:

- It is too cold out—I have used this one
- It is too hot out—I have used this one
- It is too humid out—I have used this one
- I don't have the right shoes—never tried this one

- I do not have the right equipment—I just never bought the equipment

- I don't have the right clothes, or no time to change

- When I lose the weight I will start working out (this one amazes me—how can this be? I swear I have heard this.)

What did you say? Yes, you read that last one right. I have heard this one a lot. I am not sure where this is coming from or going to and I am sure I want to know. What I do know is the people who have given these excuses just do not want to work out and they need to be honest with themselves and say so.

No one loves to workout. I am a fanatic about my weight and I do not like working out. Although I love being outside! I love to walk, leisurely. Especially down on the beach. Stopping and picking up shells or looking at beached jellyfish. I do not like walking 4.0 miles an hour for leisure. As I am writing right now, I am thinking I need to do my walking and my body is saying "Shhhh! She is writing. You want her to get a writer's block?" What would we do without our body to protect us?

That is exactly what we do not want because the body is the first to complain (big time) when anything goes wrong. A lower weight, better eating habits, lower blood pressure, or any other number of preventive measures could, have averted sometimes whatever the affliction may be. The body does not like to admit it. It wants to be comfortable. Even at the cost of being overweight.

We have to work out. I am not sorry to have said it to you. It is for your own good. Now that I have that statement out and you hate me, great, get over it and let us move on because you know I am telling you the truth. How many overweight, happy people do you know? I mean, happy and have no complaints about their knees, the size clothes they wear, the way they look, the way people look at them or now the latest news story, the airlines making them pay for two seats? How many? If you know of someone who is happy about their overweight, I would like their name and be able to talk to them, because they do not have a reason, besides denial, to be happy. Their life is at risk.

The body works a certain way and that certain way has guidelines. The good Lord did not make a 5'2 woman's frame to carry 300 plus pounds. I am not just talking about how it looks. I am talking about the ability to function. Ask the knees! I am curious on how many knee replacements are because of overweight. I am just curious! We do not only workout so we look and feel good. That is probably half if not more of an overweight person's mental battle is their body. We then have the whole health issue that goes with that.

"I am not overweight." That is what everyone says. I said it too! When I started this lifestyle change, remember this all came about by my doctor mentioning the word diabetes in a doctor's visit. I know many people who would have shrugged it off. I know many people who have shrugged it off and chalked it up as life. I am not one of those people.

I want to be as perfect as possible, which opens a whole other idea for a book, but I do know that I do not want to be sick or afflicted because of my negligence. I want the personal responsibility. If I were to be diagnosed with Type II Diabetes, and my doctor said "It's hereditary. There's nothing you can do." I would not be happy, but at least I did not cause it. I could not have prevented it.

But, when in fact, the doctor stands there and says you have this or that and it is because of your lifestyle, and you know you could change this and that, wouldn't you want to? I wanted to. Was I happy? I was not happy before the visit because the next size I was going to have to buy was a 16. I just assumed the clothing industry was making clothes smaller. It was pure denial. I wear a 4/6 now. (Some kids 16's as well.)

I did not love eating, but I wanted to enjoy what I ate. My son now tells me I had dessert after lunch and dinner! Yuck! I have it once to twice a week now, maybe! Now where am I going with this? The food change was a start, but I had to burn off what I had already amassed. Scheduling the almighty workout into my daily schedule was not a choice. Exercise was not a choice if I wanted to lose the weight. It was mandatory.

You will now need to get your piece of paper with your goals on it. (Thought I forgot about it, didn't you?) The one we put together back in Chapter 1. Let us look at that. You have put down a schedule of daily exercise. Monday through Sunday, with a form of exercise and some amount of time allocated for each day. There should be a few rest days in there and if you did not put those in, please do so now. Rest is important.

Recommendation for your body to recoup is two days. These rest days should not be back to back. The schedule you put together for your exercise regime is only as good as the doing. (Remember - BCD and the D=do)

Of course, I need to make sure we are on the same page. (This is time for BCD time sync!) Let me reiterate—and I cannot say this enough. If you do not exercise and you do not watch your portions, do not expect to see a decrease in numbers. It does not work like that. You cannot get depressed because you know what to do. If your weight is not going down, you have obviously chosen not to "D", do the part of weight loss that is just as important as the other parts. Exercise is one of the doing parts.

In the beginning of your weight loss and lifestyle change, it is so important to exercise for thirty plus days with no interruptions to time or dates. (I hope people would know that this does not apply if you have a family emergency or such.) Why is this so important? Because you are too vulnerable and may let the days *slip away*. We do that because we are human.

It is not a big deal to say, "What will one day hurt?" Only when one day turns to two and two turns to three and before you know it, it has been a month (thirty days) with no exercise. After thirty days, *anything* becomes a habit. It does not matter if it is good or bad. If you do not exercise for thirty days, that will become your habit. (How do you think you got to where you are today?) If you workout for thirty days, that will become your habit. It is your choice. You also need to have some other exercise items in check.

Everyone knows the equation for weight loss success is to burn more than you consume. Everyone knows, but not every one does. Why do they not apply this knowledge? Because it is not fun. Exercise or watch television? The vote is in for the television! If you are a couch potato, do not eat. Unfortunately, couch potatoes and overeating go together. Why? Because when you are watching television, you are not paying attention to portion control.

Besides telling people about the need for exercise, I tell him or her to find an exercise that they like. If not love it altogether. That is so when that time comes to workout, you do not think of it that way. You think of it as playing racquetball, walking, skiing, dancing or whatever it is that you have decided for your workout.

My workouts consist of walking and aerobics. I am now looking into taking dancing lessons and wall climbing. I have also started hiking. One of my girlfriends wanted me to try Pilates because she loves it. I tried it. I did not like it. I did not even enjoy it. I knew if I decided that was to be my exercise of choice, I would not exercise. Why would I not exercise? It hurt my neck. I did not like rolling around. It was uncomfortable to me. It made me not feel well. My friend loves it and it works for her. Her choice of exercise could be my excuse for not working out.

What works for one person may not for another that is why you have to find what you like to do, and then you have to commit. Make sure that it's fun and that will help you to keep this commitment.

Reaching your cardio heart rate is an extremely important part of getting to the point of losing weight. The cardio heart rate seems to be something so hard to understand because no one understands the concepts behind taking it. However, it is not difficult. Especially, with all the optional equipment we have today. They have watches that monitor your heart rate and all you have to do is look at your "watch". However, if you did not want to buy one there is a real easy way to know if your heart rate has reached the calorie-burning zone.

After you stretch, you need to get into your warm up period, which should be about ten minutes. You will see some increase in your heart rate, but not enough to reach the calorie-burning arena. Once you are into your routine, about ten minutes (twenty minutes total with warm up) you should feel your heart beating faster and you should feel a little taxed. You should be able to keep a conversation with a little effort. If you are able to talk without any effort, you are not there yet. If you cannot even respond, you are working too hard. For the calories to come off, you need to keep this increased cardio heart rate for 30-45 minutes. Increased heart rate equates fat burn.

What do you choose for your exercise? Walk, run, tennis, golf, weight lifting, whatever it is, do it often. The point is to get off your butt. Remember the plus is you can change the exercise everyday if you wish. (I recommend changing exercise routines often). I trade off my walking off with aerobics about every six weeks because at six weeks my body (and yours) will become accustomed to the workout and does not utilize the exercise to its greatest potential. For the next six weeks, I do something else.

You can trade off between only two exercises or trade off between six. All I do is change between two. If I do not want to change the exercise, I change the speed of the walking I am doing. If it is aerobics, I change the routines I do from a medium intensity to a high intensity. This too can use different muscles and burn more calories. If you are a casual walker, take it up to the level of a power walker. That is what I do. There are many other fun exercises that maybe you have not thought of as a way to lose weight. I have pulled a few from the Ohio State University Medical Center website for you to see and ponder on. They cover all seasons. These activities each have the calories burned in 30 minutes. (Calories burned are based on a 150-pound person.)

- Trudge through the snow: 170
- Dash through the snow: 204
- Climb the stairs at a ski resort: 550
- Cross-country ski: 306
- Return holiday gifts: 85
- Plant a winter indoor garden: 61
- Stack firewood: 206
- Go sledding: 238
- Build a snowman: 119
- Play basketball: 200
- Play hockey: 465
- Have a snowball fight: 272
- Make snow angels: 154
- Ice skate: 238
- Swim: 250

As you can see many of these are winter items because after the holidays, that is the prime time we gain the most weight. However, there are many fun ways throughout the year to get that weight off without thinking about it.

If you find something you love to do for your exercise time, and you look forward to it, boredom should not be a problem. Make sure, if you are even approaching the thought of "aw—this again…" change your exercise. There are so many awesome types of exercise to choose from with or without tapes or equipment. I was just at a store the other day and they had exercise tapes ranging from belly dancing to hip-hop and beyond! Get your booty grooving!

If you happen to live in a warm client (which I do not—yet) your sources of exercise are unlimited. Volleyball, walking, hiking, biking, tennis, jogging and the list goes on and on, year-round! If you live in a colder climate, you will have to get creative. If you are financially able to, a gym is always a great investment as they have unlimited resources. If joining a health club is not a feasible option that does not mean you cannot access one. Make it a point to go and "check it out" once a year. Most clubs will give you a two-week trial membership.

During the cold months if the weather is not horrendous, you can still do some exercises outside. I know I walked outside last year until late October. I start walking outside again in early April. I get out half of the year, but there are those few sporadic days during the year that we get freaky weather and the weather is cooperative. Like a sixty-two degree-day in February. Go out and walk!

Just remember the point is if you get out of the habit of exercising for thirty days it is just like when you started. It will not be a habit and you will have to retrain yourself to stay on the mark. So do not miss more than two workouts in a row. I realize that life can hand you some real tough plays in life, but the results of not working out can be for life.

For those of you who have not worked out in sometime (or at all), it will be an effort to get back into the swing. If you are starting for the first time, I would suggest you try to find a friend with whom you can workout. It is fun to workout with someone because you can talk and talk and before you know it the time is up and you sometimes wish there was more time remaining so you could keep talking with your friend.

Friends can be an instrumental part of your success to working out. When making the decision on whom that will be, you need to consider their level of commitment to the exercise regime or your willingness to go on without them if they were to renege. I had this happen to me several times, many years ago. My son was in kindergarten and I wanted to get rid of the remaining baby fat. We had moved to a new neighborhood and I had found a neighbor who was looking for someone to walk with. That was great!

For the first few weeks, everything went great. Then week by week, she would call with one reason or another on why she could not walk. When it got down to one day a week, I realized I needed to go on without her. That is what I did. Then I found another friend who lived by my son's school. The same thing occurred. The first few weeks were awesome and then week by week, something would come up and it resulted in maybe walking once a month, if I were lucky. Once again, I went solo.

When you start working out—this is usually the time your body will let you know any and everything that is wrong, as a ploy, hopefully to stop your success. Listen to your body, but do not baby it. Do not give into fake symptoms. If you are running a fever, do not work out. If you are puking, do not workout. If you have a serious injury, do not work out. However, if you have dull aches and pains and they have been there forever, your doctor has told you they are nothing to worry about, get off your butt and on with your exercise.

About three quarters of the way into my training for a marathon last year my left knee starting hurting. I do not mean aching I mean ripping and tearing. I have a high tolerance for pain, so I let it go for a while. After another two months, I had to see the doctor.

After many tests had been performed, and the results read, nothing was revealed. But, on seeing a sports doctor, he discovered my left leg was 1/8" longer than the right, thus the pains I was feeling were real, but they were adjustment pains. However, I knew the pain was not anything I had ever felt before and I did not want to make a lifelong injury. However, I never stopped working out! Now when my knee hurts I just keep walking with the promise when I get home I will take some anti-inflammatory medication, or I slow it down. Usually I do not even need that. The cool down gives my knee time to recoup.

Remember that anything done for 30 days becomes a habit, but unfortunately (think about the New Year's Resolutions) people do not go much beyond 14-21 days. Why do people give up so easily? It is too much effort. It is not seeing the changes fast enough. There is never enough time and people are always too tired. I am tired right now but I know as soon as I finish with my writing this evening I am hitting the treadmill. I have to do it for me.

Another pothole (sounds like Chicago in the spring!) in your weight loss journey is the alternative plans to your workout if you are unable to do what you had planned. Let me explain. I live in Chicago. Need I say anything more about the weather? The weather is unpredictable. (This week alone it has been 80 for two days and 50 for three). I have planned to walk the local track every day between three and four. I go to my sister's, park my car and away I go. The weather, with the different seasons, sometimes has other plans for me.

In the summertime, they do not spray the track for mosquitoes because the track runs through a forest preserve. In the winters, it can be dangerous depending on snowfall or ice. The springs and falls can bring violent thunderstorms, which are unsafe conditions in which to walk. What is my alternative? I walk in the house (by means of treadmill or DVD) or do aerobics. Years ago, I bought two-mile walking DVD's I can do in the house and when I cannot go outside because of the weather, I walk in the house. I also have recently purchased a treadmill so I can walk more miles. The treadmill also gives a little variety with the different programs, cardio or fat-burn.

Balance what you eat with how often you exercise. Less exercise means less burn that means less eats. "So if I exercise more can I eat more?" No. If you exercise more and continue to eat what you are suppose to, guess what will happen? You will lose weight! Is this not what this it is all about? You cannot eat a five-course meal, go lie on the couch for four hours, get up and go to bed and wonder why in the morning your scale has increased by three pounds!

Remember I told you earlier that you have to view food as a fuel. You must burn what goes in or it gets stored. Storing equates fat and that is what this whole lifestyle change is about, getting rid of the fat. I ran across a fraction layout on the website webmd.com that was eye opening and very encouraging. It would be well worth your time to type it up and put it in your workout room. The fraction is the 80/20 fraction.

- 80= exercise regular and eat well
- 20 = slip due to work schedule or holidays

None of us are perfect. It is good to know and good to see that if we slip, the slip is not what matters, but if and how often we get back up. We cannot slip 80% of the time, with 20% of the time keeping it together and then gripe because the weight is not going anywhere. It will not.

One of the wonders of the human body is that it does not take a whole lot to burn a few more calories. Let us take walking. You will burn calories just by walking, but by simply adding arm movements, you can burn even more. Biking is another. You can start out on the easy gear and either change gears to add more resistance or change the scene by adding hills. Once again, remember, more resistance, more burn.

One of the older exercises that never loses its popularity and burns an extreme amount of calories is weight lifting. By adding more weight, you will increase the burn rate. Doing other little tweaks to your exercise routine can increase the burn rate. Be creative. As you increase your workouts (because you will) try to avoid overdoing it. An example is walking with weights. Walking with weights is bad on joints. It will help burn a few more calories, but the injuries this could cause far outweigh the advantages. If you want to burn more, swing your arms more or increase your pace.

Once you have your ways set in your exercise routine, you will find you will want to reward yourself with extracurricular exercise events. Find fun events like minimarathons. I heard your scream. I know it sounds like exercise, but these can be a lot of fun. I have participated in several and I will be doing another one this year. Besides being with other people and having fun, it gives you a picture of where you are health wise. Several years ago, when I did my first 2.5 I thought it would be a breeze, until at least a dozen senior citizens finished before me! How embarrassing! These extracurricular exercise events are good for calibration on where you are and how you need to adjust. A 2.5 minimarathon should be a breeze if you are walking 3.0 miles a day. If it is not, maybe you are not doing that much. There is usually a health fair that accompany these events, where you can get samples of new products and ideas for other exercise ideas.

Let us talk about the pluses to exercising. I know I can lose weight, keep my blood sugar down and my blood pressure down, but are there not any perks? (As if those were not enough.) Here is a big plus to exercising! Everyone knows working out helps stress. How many times have we heard this? I have had many people tell me that working out causes their stress!

Well then, you have not found an exercise you love. Remember you need to look forward to it.

Exercising decreases stress. I know there are times I am so upset with my son or husband that when I get on the treadmill I mentally think I am running away from them! After working out (walking) for an hour and getting in tune with my body, I have well forgotten or at least reduced the tension that I had before starting my workout.

Working out can take that negative energy and put it to use in a positive way. If you are into boxing, well that says it for its self. Any exercise that spends energy will take your stress level down several levels. I also have found that I do not get upset as fast as I use to. I could attribute this to a better self-esteem, but I know that I do not want to rip people's heads off all the time. I am much more calm and collective.

"I have read everything you have written, but I still don't like to exercise. I'll watch what I eat but that's it!" Well that may be so but here are two tidbits for you to chew on while you are on the couch.

According to the National Institutes of Study, couch potatoes are 2.5 times more likely to develop dementia than regular exercisers. In addition, brisk walking or biking at least 30 minutes, five times each week can help improve insulin sensitivity—remember I talked about the glycemic index? So if you do not like to exercise these may be facts that will encourage you to workout.

As I stated before your exercise regime should be along these lines: heart specialists' recommendations are 45-60 minutes to lose weight, 4-5 times a week and 30 minutes 3-4 days a week to maintain. If you are in the 45-60 minutes, to lose weight you have to increase your heart rate into a weight loss zone. You cannot walk 45-60 minutes at a snail's pace and expect to lose weight. The walking is great no matter whom you are and no matter what speed you walk, but the weight loss results of your walking will vary depending on the speed you maintain. Your heart rate is how this is determined. (See Appendix B).

There are exercises that do not increase your heart rate to a weight loss rate. You want to avoid these in the early part of your lifestyle change. You could add them in later with other exercises. And of course with the start of any physical activity you are not used to, please check with your doctor before beginning your new exercise routine.

Earlier in the book, I said I would talk about your exercise time being a "sacred time". When I first started working out (walking or aerobics) in the house because of the inclement and always-changing Chicago weather, people would constantly interrupt me. After the first week or so, there was no end in sight to the interruptions. I told everyone who were involved, I was not to be interrupted between three and four o'clock because I was working out. For a few days, the interruptions kept up but I refused to talk to anyone. I gave them "the look" and I never answered the phone or doorbell. That was my time and I wanted to lose weight so bad no one was going to stop me. Besides, it was clear to me those involved did not think I was serious about losing weight. Now, today, everyone knows if I am working out, I will not answer the phone, I will not answer the door, and I will not talk to any person who needs a piece of my exercise time.

In any exercise program there is always a chance that injury could occur. What happens if you are injured? What happens to the workout schedule you have so diligently put together and have been faithful to? If you have the unfortunate event of being injured do not just up and quit your workouts. This is where most people miss the mark.

An injury does not mean your lifestyle change is over. Call your doctor and see what exercise can replace your regular exercise. If the injury is serious enough that your doctor says no go on physical activity then the solution is to just rest. If that is what is called for then that is what you need to do. An injured body does you no-good. If you need to change days to rest, make sure you do it. Saying I will do it on Thursday means nothing if on Thursday, you do nothing.

Life is sometimes unpredictable and can consume days and before you know it, it is a week later. Adjust your workouts to be able to have "the quantity" needed. However, if a situation arises where a large amount of time is needed to step away, continue to watch your portions and pick up on your exercise regime as soon as you can.

6

It's All About You!

Let us wrap this up so you can get started. This chapter is my cheerleading chapter. You need to decide to lose weight. You need to want to lose weight. You need to put in action those decisions you know will help you to carry out your weight loss goal. I think you now know there is no secret to losing weight. It is all in the self-control realm.

You need to decide how you are going to accomplish it, which I have showed you how to do; you just need to insert the specifics. (It is not your lifestyle if I put in every detail for you. I have to let you make some choices!) You are the one who needs to put your mind to doing it and GO AND DO IT! (I am good, but not that good.) Unless you hire a personal trainer who will live with you, no one is going to be breathing down your neck. No one is going to be policing your plates for serving sizes. No one is going to be standing in your living room with their hands on their hips, foot tapping and asking you why you are not working out. This whole lifestyle change requires self-discipline.

Remember it is all about you. You need to be determined and remind yourself monthly, weekly, daily and hourly it is for you. If you do not do it, no one will. Make little signs and put them up around the house in spots you frequent. Tell yourself you can do it. Remind yourself there are x amount of pounds left before success is yours. Write down the next reward and put a picture next to it. Several companies make motivational posters that you can buy to motivate yourself. Do whatever you need to do to help you carry out this lifestyle change. It is all for you. The purpose is to make you look better, feel better and live longer.

This lifestyle change is about you. It is for you. It will benefit only you! (There's a good chance your significant other will appreciate the results too.) I am not into myself unless it comes to my health and my health is the only area that is a direct result of my eating and exercise behavior. If I watch what I eat, work my body as I am suppose to then I will see results. That also applies on the other side if I do not eat right or workout I will see the results. The weight will not leave.

Heart disease, diabetes, obesity, knee problems, hip problems, respiratory problems could be mine if I do not keep everything in line. I am not speaking negatively, that is just how it is. If I sow a sedentary, overeating lifestyle, I reap a fat me. If I am insistent about my portion sizes of what I consume and I am active, then I reap a healthy me. It is my choice.

A thought came to me when I started this whole lifestyle change. I am very meticulous about my car. Oil change at 3000, my tank rarely goes below a quarter tank. I keep it washed and clean inside and out and if I get a flat tire, I feel like someone hurt a relative! But, here is what I discovered. I take care of my car like that and I do not even live in it! Wow! What a wake up call!

We put bad stuff in our body (we would never think about putting water in our gas tanks although that is cheaper than gas, because our car would not run on water and it would ruin the engine). So why do we put junk food in our bodies? We talked about that. We need to think about that. We need to meditate on that. If we ate right and exercised, we would feel better. That's a given.

Just losing a few pounds does so much to the psyche of a person. When you start seeing the results of everything you put into practice, it sends you to the moon! Your self-esteem sharply increases. You feel better, you look better and now you even like yourself! I have so far failed to see anything bad about losing weight. Have you? I have never seen a person who has lost weight, bummed out; going around saying, "I look horrible. I'd feel better if I didn't look so good."

"What if I get depressed during this lifestyle change?" Depression is not in the equation if you are following the rules, because you will have success. There is no reason to get depressed at plateaus. We have addressed those. Remember those are—temporary. If you are not having success in losing weight with your new lifestyle, you probably are not following the rules and the emotion you should then have is anger. Get angry with yourself. Grow up! Take control of your life!

I know of several people who when they get depressed they eat. All I can say is, do not eat for emotional reasons. I know that is a real problem for people which I cannot empathize with, but please do not do it. It is not worth it. You will eat because you get depressed, but then once you are done eating, you will be depressed because you did what you know you were not suppose to. It is a vicious cycle.

You have already identified the problem of eating because of emotions in most cases, so find some other vent for the depression. You must get creative and trade off eating for exercise. If you do not like exercise, even the ones you picked, the threat alone of exercise may ward off any bouts of depression. This is where the buddy system can come in handy. When you feel like eating pick up the phone. Call someone who will encourage you and remind you of why you decided to make this lifestyle change and why you should stay on course.

One of the many steps to failure in this weight loss and lifestyle change is taking too big of steps. Little steps get you farther. You can adjust better and faster with little steps. When I am walking, I do not try to walk the steps my six-foot husband takes. I would probably get hurt and if I did make it I would be sore and discouraged because it took too much work and it was not fun.

A weight loss/lifestyle change can be fun. Try new foods. There are so many different fruits and veggies out there—and oh, the creations that can be made with turkey! And it does not stop at my house. I can eat out and have a turkey burger! I was ecstatic when I found out that my son's favorite burger place had turkey burgers! Bring on the burgers! (Make sure there are lots of lettuce, tomatoes and onions.)

You need to see food as your fuel and not as a means of venting. Does this mean no dessert? No. Portion is the sole objective. Have the brownie. Make sure it is in correct proportion to the portion stated on the package. Have a cookie. Make sure the portion is what is stated on the package. Most of all remember, make sure it is within your daily allowable intake. You cannot have those yummies if you used all of your calories and carbs for breakfast, lunch and dinner. Remember the trade-offs. You will get good at this as time goes on. Trust me. I am a brownie freak.

Try new exercise. The more you put into anything the more you get out of it. One of my objectives when I loss weight was to walk a marathon. I loss the weight. I trained for a marathon. I walked a half marathon, which is 13.2 miles, for you nonmarathoners. So why am I telling you that? I pushed myself to a new level.

I knew there was never going to be a day I would purposely walk farther than five miles. Five miles is a lot, but I needed a reason to do more. (Are you surprised I am human?) The training for a marathon is intense. (I trained for a full marathon, but then I had an injury and my doctor said I should only do a half.) It was hard training. I discovered muscles that I cannot even find on diagrams!

My point is that I have made my body do more and it was something new. After I had finished the marathon, I decided I would like to take up hiking. I have also looked into rock climbing. If you keep it new and fresh you are more likely to be ambitious about wanting to try different activities, and in turn, you are working out and loving it!

Always make sure, when you reach a goal you reward yourself. (Do not reward yourself with anything eatable!) You deserve it. I talked with my old coach once and was telling her about this book, and talked about the reward system. She got a big smile on her face and said, "I know! I am going to go and buy a fireplace today because I reached my weight goal!" I had not said anything to her previously about the reward system in weight loss. She discovered the value of rewarding herself.

Constantly remind yourself why you are doing this weight loss and life-style change. Have your paper in front of you and make copies if you need to. Hang it everywhere. You need to have the reason imbedded in you. When your body gets tired or you feel like "buffeting" it for dinner—look at your paper. Look at your journal. See where you were and where you have gone. Can you afford it weight wise? Sometimes you can, with self-control and portion control. Sometimes you can't.

Seeing the numbers is sometimes all it takes to stay on track. Pictures are good too. As the weight starts rolling off take pictures of the new you and put them up where you can see them. Remember a longer life and a happier you is the result of all this hard work. Do it for you!

Keep going. Do not let this weight loss and lifestyle change be "for awhile". When I started losing large amounts of weight and I was down to a size eight (that was then; I am now a size four.) I was buying new clothes. A woman I worked with, said to me "Don't get rid of your fat clothes!" I could not believe it. That mind-set is what keeps her from losing the weight. When you start dropping the weight, buy new clothes and immediately get rid of the old. Do not give yourself any inlet for not losing the weight. Do it for you! Just knowing you have no clothes to wear, if you were to gain the weight back, could be enough incentive to not going back to your old eating ways.

Your size is about you. What is your ideal (realistic) size? Mine was an eight—I am now at a 4/6. Aim, reach and achieve. It is all about you. It is your look. What do you want to gain in all this? A smaller butt? Stronger legs? Aim, reach and achieve. After accomplishing all of this, how do you want to feel physically? Do you want your back to stop hurting? Do you want your knees to stop whining? Do you want to be able to climb four steps and not be ready to drop-dead? There is only good that will come out of this lifestyle change. Aim, reach and achieve. B-C-D. Believe, commit and do.

I do not even know you and I believe in you. The least you can do for you is to believe in you. If you are not strong enough, make sure you get a friend to do this with you. It is fun to have someone there to cheerlead for you when you are getting upset or when the nasty scale is hanging onto a number that should have been gone weeks before. It is good to have someone to talk you out of going out and getting the biggest hot fudge sundae because work sucked.

If your significant other is unable to be your cheerleader, find someone who you can call whenever the going gets rough. Do not pick the friend who is a nurse, and works twenty-three hours a day. She will not be available for you. Find someone who you can talk to pretty much whenever. Unfortunately, I did not have anyone. I found the inner strength to keep driving myself. Remember I wanted it bad enough to make a change and I believe you do to.

Give me a D. Give me an O. Give me a N. Give me a T. Give me a G. Give me an I. Give me a V. Give me an E. Give me an U. Give me a P. What does that spell? DON'T GIVE UP! You go! DON'T GIVE UP! You live, love and be happy with you! Celebrate life. Celebrate your new eating habits. You need to believe you can do it. B-C-D. Believe, Commit and Do. Remember it is all about you!

APPENDIX A

These are the recommended serving sizes as stated in the American Diabetes Association Exchange List for Meal Planning. Each item would count as 15 grams of carbohydrates, or 1 carb.

Most condiments are counted as "free foods" as long as you stay within the serving size on the package.

Breads

Bagel, 4 oz.	4 oz.
Bread Crumbs, dried	3 Tbsp.
Bread Crumbs, fresh	1/2 cup
Croutons, low fat	1 cup
English Muffin	1/2
Hamburger or Hot Dog Bun	1/2 (1 oz.)
Pita Bread, 6 inches across	1/2 (1 oz.)
Raisin Bread (unfrosted)	1 slice (1 oz.)
Reduced—calorie bread	2 slices
Roll, plain, small	1 (1 oz.)
Rye or Pumpernickel Bread	1 slice (1 oz.)
Tortilla, corn, flour, 6 inches across	1
Tortilla, flour, 10 inches across	1/2
Waffle, 4 inch square, reduced-fat	1

Pasta/Grains

Bulgar (cooked)	1/2 cup
Cornmeal (dry)	3 Tbsp.
Cornstarch (dry)	2 Tbsp.
Couscous (cooked)	1/3 cup
Flour (dry)	3 Tbsp.
Kasha (cooked)	1/2 cup
Millet (cooked)	1/3 cup
Pasta (cooked)	1/3 cup
Rice, white or brown (cooked)	1/3 cup

Crackers and Snacks

Animal Crackers	8
Bread sticks, crisp, 4 in. long x 1/2 in.	2 (2/3 oz.)

White Bread (French and Italian)	1 slice	Graham Crackers, 2 1/2 in. square	3
Whole Wheat Bread	1 slice	Matzoh	3/4 oz.
		Melba Toast	4 slices
		Oyster crackers	24
		Popcorn (popped, no added fat, or low fat Microwave)	3 cups
Cereals			
Bran Cereals	1/2 cup	Pretzels	3/4 cup
Cereals, unsweetened	3/4 cup	Rice cakes, 4 inches across	2
Granola, low fat	1/4 cup	Rice cakes, 1 1/2 inches across	8
Grape-Nuts®	1/4 cup	Rye wafers (crisp) 2 in. x 3 1/2 in.	2
Grits (cooked)	1/2 cup	Saltine type crackers	6
Hot cereal (cooked)	1/2 cup	Snack chips, fat-free (tortilla, potato)	15-20
Shredded Wheat	1/2 cup	Whole Wheat Crackers (no added fat)	2-5

Starchy Vegetables		**Starchy Foods Prepared with Fat**	
Baked Beans	1/3 cup	Biscuit, 2 1/2 inches across	1
Corn	1/2 cup	Chow Mein Noodles	1/2 cup
Corn on the cob, large	1/2 (5 oz.)	Cornbread, 2 inch cube	1 (2 oz.)
Mixed veg w/corn, peas or pasta	1 cup	Crackers, round, butter type	6
Peas, Green	1/2 cup	Croutons	1 cup
Plantain	1/2 cup	French fries, oven baked	1 cup

Potato, baked with skin	1/4 large	Granola	1/4 cup
Potato, boiled or mashed	1/2 cup	Hummus	1/3 cup
Pumpkin	3/4 cup	Muffin, 5 oz.	1/5 (1 oz.)
Squash, winter (acorn, butternut)	1 cup	Pancake, 4 inches across	1
Yam, sweet potato, plain	1/2 cup	Popcorn, microwave	3 cups
		Sandwich crackers with cheese of peanut butter filling	3
		Stuffing, bread, prepared	1/3 cup
Dried Beans, Peas and Lentils		Taco Shell, 6 inches across	2
Beans and Peas (cooked)	1/2 cup	Waffle, 4 inch square	1
Lentils (cooked)	1/2 cup	Whole Wheat Crackers, fat added	4-6
Lima Beans (cooked)	2/3 cup		

Fruit

Apple, unpeeled, small	1 (4 oz.)	Papaya	1 cup cubes
Apples, dried	4 rings	Peach, medium, fresh	1
Applesauce, unsweetened	1/2 cup	Peaches, canned	1/2 cup
			1/2
Apricots, fresh	4 whole	Pear, large, fresh	
Apricots, dried	8 halves	Pears, canned	1/2 cup
Apricots, canned	1/2 cup	Pineapple, fresh	3/4 cup
Banana, small	1 (4 oz.)	Pineapple, canned	1/2 cup
Blackberries	3/4 cup	Plums, small	2
Blueberries	3/4 cup	Plums, canned	1/2 cup
Cantaloupe, small	1 cup cubes	Plums, dried (prunes)	3

Casaba melon	1 cup cubes	Raisins	2 Tbsp.
Cherries, sweet, fresh	12	Raspberries	1 cup
Cherries, sweet, canned	1/2 cup	Strawberries, whole berries	1 1/4 cup
Currants	2 Tbsp.	Tangerine, small	2
Dates	3	Watermelon, sliced	1
Figs, fresh, large	1.5		
Figs, fresh, medium	2		
Figs, dried	1.5	**Fruit Juice**	
Fruit Cocktail	1/2 cup	Apple Juice/Cider	1/2 cup
Grapefruit, large	1/2	Cranberry juice cocktail	1/3 cup
Grapefruit, sections, canned	3/4 cup	Cranberry juice cocktail, reduced-calorie	1 cup
Grapes, small	17	Fruit juice blends, 100% juice	1/3 cup
Guava, medium	1	Grape Juice	1/3 cup
Honeydew melon	1 cup cubes	Grapefruit Juice	1/2 cup
Kiwi	1	Orange Juice	1/2 cup
Mandarin Oranges, canned	3/4 cup	Pineapple Juice	1/2 cup
Mango, small	1/2 cup	Prune Juice	1/3 cup
Nectarine, small	1		
Orange, small	1		
		Reduced-fat Milk	
		2% milk	1 cup
		Evaporated low fat (2%) milk	1/2 cup
Fat-Free and Low Fat Milk		Soy milk	1 cup
Fat- Free (skim) milk	1 cup	Sweet acidophilus milk	1 cup
1/2 % milk	1 cup	Yogurt (plain, low-fat)	3/4 cup
1% milk	1 cup		

Buttermilk, fat-free or low fat	1 cup		
Evaporated fat-free milk	1/2 cup		
Fat-free dry milk	1/3 cup dry	**Food**	
Soy milk, fat-free or low fat	1 cup	Milk, chocolate, whole	1 cup
Yogurt	2/3 cup	Pie, fruit, 2 crusts	1/6 pie
		Pie, Pumpkin or custard	1/8 pie
		Potato chips, snack chips	12 -18
Whole Milk		Pudding, any kind	1/2 cup
		Reduced-calorie meal replacement shake	1 can
Whole Milk	1 cup		
Evaporated whole milk	1/2 cup	Salad dressing, fat-free	1/4 cup
Goat's milk	1 cup	Sherbet, sorbet	1/2 cup
Kefir	1 cup	Spaghetti or pasta sauce, canned	1/2 cup
Yogurt (plain, made from whole milk)	3/4 cup	Sports drinks	1 cup
		Sugar	1 Tbsp.
		Sweet Roll or Danish, 2 1/2 oz.	1
Food		Syrup, light	1/4 cup
Angel food cake, unfrosted	1/12 cake	Syrup, regular	2 Tbsp.
Brownie, small, unfrosted	2 inch square	Tortilla Chips	6-12
Cake, unfrosted	2 inch square	Vanilla Wafers	5
Cake, frosted	2 inch square	Yogurt, frozen	1/2 cup
Cookie, sugar-free, small	3	Yogurt, frozen, fat-free	1/3 cup
Cookie, sugar-free, large	1	Yogurt, low fat with fruit	1 cup
Cookie with cream filling, small	2		
Cupcake, frosted, small	1		

		Moderate Use	
Cranberry sauce, jellied	1/4 cup		
Donut, plain cake, medium	1	Cream cheese, fat-free	1 Tbsp.
Energy, sort or breakfast bar	1	Creamers, nondairy, liquid	1 Tbsp.
Fruit juice bars, frozen, 100% juice	1	Creamers, nondairy, powdered	2 tsp.
Fruit snacks, chewy, fruit concentrate	1 roll	Mayonnaise, fat-free	1 Tbsp.
Fruit spreads, 100% fruit	1 1/2 Tbsp.	Mayonnaise, reduced-fat	1 tsp.
Gelatin, regular	1/2 cup	Margarine, fat-free	4 Tbsp.
Gingersnaps	3	Margarine, reduced-fat	1 tsp.
Granola bar or snack bar	1	Salad dressing, fat-free	1 Tbsp.
Honey	1 Tbsp.	Salad dressing, fat-free, Italian	2 Tbsp.
Ice-Cream (any kind)	1/2 cup	Salsa	1/4 cup
Jam or jelly, regular	1 Tbsp.	Sour Cream, fat-free, reduced-fat	1 Tbsp.
		Whipped Topping, light or fat-free	2 Tbsp.
		Whipped Topping, regular	1 Tbsp.
Fat Foods		Candy, hard, sugar-free	1
		Jam or jelly, low sugar or light	2 tsp.
Avocado, medium	2 Tbsp.	Syrup, sugar-free	2 Tbsp.
Oil (canola, olive, peanut)	1 tsp.	Ketchup	1 Tbsp.
Olives, ripe, black, large	8	Pickles, Dill, large	1 1/2
Olives, green, stuffed, large	10	Taco Sauce	1 Tbsp.
Nuts (almonds, cashews)	6	Soy Sauce, regular or light	1 Tbsp.
Nuts, mixed (50% peanuts)	6	Cocoa Powder, unsweetened	1 Tbsp.
Nuts, peanuts	10		

Nuts, pecans	4 halves	Cranberries or rhubarb, sweetened w/sugar subs	1/2 cup
Peanut Butter (smooth or crunchy)	1/2 Tbsp.		
Sesame Seeds	1 Tbsp.	**Vegetables**	
Tahini Paste	2 tsp.	NonStarch, raw	1 cup
Margarine, stick, tub or squeeze	1 tsp.	NonStarch, cooked	1/2 cup
Margarine, lower-fat	1 Tbsp.	Avocado, medium	2 Tbsp.
Mayonnaise, regular	1 tsp.	Dried beans, peas, lentils (cooked)	1/2 cup
Mayonnaise, reduced-fat	1 Tbsp.		
Nuts, walnuts, English	4 halves		
Oil (corn, safflower, soy-bean)	1 tsp.	**Meats**	
Salad dressing, regular	1 Tbsp.	Turkey, white meat, no skin	1 oz.
Salad dressing, reduced-fat	2 Tbsp.	Cod, fresh and frozen	1 oz.
Seeds (pumpkin, sunflower)	1 Tbsp.	Haddock, fresh and frozen	1 oz.
Bacon, cooked	1 slice	Trout, fresh and frozen	1 oz.
Bacon, grease	1 tsp.	Lox	1 oz.
Butter, stick	1 tsp.	Crab	1 oz.
Butter, whipped	2 tsp.	Scallops	1 oz.
Butter, reduced-fat	1 Tbsp.	Shellfish	1 oz.
Chitterlings, boiled	2 Tbsp.	Pheasant, no skin	1 oz.
Coconut, sweetened, shredded	2 Tbsp.	Buffalo	1 oz.
Cream, half-and-half	2 Tbsp.	Beef, lean, trimmed of fat	1 oz.
Cream Cheese, regular	1 Tbsp.	Fresh Ham	1 oz.
Cream Cheese, reduced-fat	1 1/2 Tbsp.	Canadian Bacon	1 oz.

Shortening or Lard	1 tsp.	Pork, center loin chop	1 oz.
Sour Cream, regular	2 Tbsp.	Veal, lean chop, roast	1 oz.
Sour Cream, reduced-fat	3 Tbsp.	Salmon, fresh or canned	1 oz.
		Sardines, canned, medium	2
		Goose, no skin	1 oz.
Meats		Beef, ground, meat loaf, corned beef, short ribs	1 oz.
Chicken, white or dark meat, no skin	1 oz.	Lamb, rib roast, ground	1 oz.
Cornish Hen, no skin	1 oz.	Chicken, dark or white, with skin	1 oz.
Flounder, fresh and frozen	1 oz.	Chicken, fried with skin	1 oz.
Halibut, fresh and frozen	1 oz.	Pork, spareribs	1 oz.
Tune, fresh or canned in water	1 oz.	Pork, sausage	1 oz.
Clams	1 oz.	Pork, ground pork	1 oz.
Lobster	1 oz.	Duck, no skin	1 oz.
Shrimp	1 oz.	Venison	1 oz.
Ostrich	1 oz.	Tuna, canned, in oil, drained	1 oz.
Lean pork	1 oz.	Pork, top loin, Boston butt, cutlet	1 oz.
Ham, cured, canned or boiled	1 oz.	Veal Cutlet, ground or cubed, plain	1 oz.
Pork Tenderloin	1 oz.	Turkey, dark meat, skin	1 oz.
Lamb, roast, chop, leg	1 oz.	Turkey, ground with skin	1 oz.
Oysters, medium	6	Chicken, ground with skin	1 oz.
Catfish	1 oz.	Fish, fried, any product	1 oz.
Rabbit, no skin	1 oz.		

Appendix B

Target Heart Rate
(Provided by International Fitness Association)
www.ifafitness.com

AGE	60%–70%		70%–80%	
	Beats/min	Beats/10 sec	Beats/min	Beats/10 sec
To 19	121–141	20–24	141–161	24–27
20–24	119–139	20–23	139–158	23–26
25–29	116–135	19–23	135–154	23–26
30–34	113–132	19–22	132–150	22–25
35–39	110–128	18–21	128–146	21–24
40–44	107–125	18–21	125–142	21–24
45–49	104–121	17–20	121–138	20–23
50–54	101–118	17–20	118–134	20–22
55–59	98–114	16–19	114–130	19–22
60–64	95–111	16–19	111–126	19–21
65–69	92–107	15–18	107–122	18–20
70–74	89–104	15–17	104–118	17–20
75–79	86–100	14–17	100–114	17–19
80–84	83–97	16–18	97–110	16–18
85+	81–95	14–16	95–108	16–18

Checking a pulse is the easy way to determine heart rate. Your resting heart rate should be counted for 60 seconds. Counting a resting pulse rate in less time increases the chance of error. During exercise you can use 6 or 10 second pulse checks. If the pulse is counted for 6 seconds, multiply by 10 to get the heart rate in beats per minute. If the 10-second count is used, multiply by 6 to get beats per minute.

Two easy methods can be used when checking your pulse rate. One method checks the pulse at the wrist, called the radial pulse, and the other is at the neck, called the carotid pulse.

For a RADIAL PULSE CHECK, use the tips of your index and middle finger. The radial artery can be found on the thumb side of either one of your wrists. It lies just a little below the base of the thumb. The pulsing of the artery will be felt when your fingers are in the right place. Hold gently. Digital watches or those with second hands can be used. After locating the radial pulse, begin your count with "zero" on the starting time mark; then count the pulses for the desired time length.

The CAROTID PULSE CHECK is taken in a place just below the jaw along the windpipe and along the throat. Use the fingertips of the index and middle fingers to press gently. Do not move your fingers around in a massaging motion while trying to find your carotid pulse. This can lower your blood pressure and cause dizziness. The same counting systems used for the radial pulse check can be used for the carotid pulse check.

When taking your pulse check always stop exercising before beginning to count. Check your pulse quickly. Do not wait even a few seconds to rest before beginning to count. If this happens, the pulse rate will not be accurate. Resume exercising immediately after the pulse check so your heart rate does not have time to slow down out of your training heart rate range.

APPENDIX C

Two Week exert taken Angie's from personal log
Remember the info must be accurate

Date	Time	Wt.	Time	BP1	BP2	Ex.	Time	BS	Notes
9/7/04	6:30a	152.5	8:17a	114/82	110/77	55 min. walk	8:15a	119	1 hr. 10 min. Bkft
9/8/04	5:00a	153				none			Dr. appt.
9/9/04	6:30a	152				55 min walk			
9/10/04	6:00a	152.5				50 min walk			
9/11/04	6:00a	151.5	7:02a	121/81	112/80	Shopping	7:30a	136	1 hr. bkft
									Ate in 8 minutes
									Oats, fruit, sugar
9/12/04	6:00a	152				none			
9/13/04	6:30a	152.5	7:36a	117/77		50 min walk	12:50p	129	1 hr. lunch
9/14/04	6:30a	153.5				50 min walk			
9/15/04	6:30a	152.5				55 min walk			
9/16/04	6:30a	151.5	9:19a	120/72		55 min walk	9:15p	100	1 hr. dinner
9/17/04	5:30a	151.5				55 min walk			
9/18/04	6:30a	150.5							
9/19/04	6:30a	151.5	4:36p	107/76			8:05a	135	1 hr. bkft, Int Cof
9/20/04	6:30a	149				55 min walk			

- WT=weight, BP=blood pressure, Ex=exercise, BS= blood sugar
- The monitoring of blood sugar went to 3 times each week
- The days where no workout occurred were Saturdays and Sundays

- In the notes it was important to know how long after I ate did I test the blood sugar

- There are two spots for BP so if the first one was high I would wait about five minutes and then retake my BP

On 9/7/04: you can see in the notes the time that elapsed before BS was taken.

On 9/8/04: in the exercise portion I put *none* in the exercise. I made a note so that I knew I had not exercised and had not "forgotten to write it down".

On 9/11/04: notes in the note section refer to what I ate because of the reading I received when I took my BS.

On 9/14/04: I gained weight. It could be attributed to the time in the evening I ate dinner the night before, but because I didn't make a note of that I don't know why the weight went up.

There is no such thing as too much information when you are maintaining a weight loss log. As you continue to keep the log you made add sections as you see fit.

APPENDIX D

Proportionate visual sizes

SERVINGS	VISUAL SIZE
One piece of fruit or potato	About the size of a regular (60 watt) light bulb
One-half cup of vegetables	The size of a light bulb
½ cup	About the size of a racquetball
One cup of pasta	The size of a tennis ball
¾ cup	The size of a tennis ball
1 fruit serving	The size of a tennis ball
½ cup canned fruit	The size of a tennis ball
1 medium fruit	The size of a tennis ball
1 ½–2 oz cheese	Tube of lipstick or 3.5" computer disk
3 oz. meat/poultry/fish	Deck of cards or cassette tape
2 Tablespoons peanut butter	Golf ball
1 bagel	Hockey puck
Medium potato	Computer mouse
One teaspoon of peanut butter	One dice

Bibliography

Published Sources

"Risk Factors You Can Control or Treat". American Heart Association. Reproduced with permission. www.americanheartassociation. © 2006, American Heart Association, Inc.

Haas, Elson Dr., MD. Staying Healthy With Nutrition, The Complete Guide to Diet & Nutritional Medicine. 1992: 83-150

"The Meals Exchange List". The Exchange Lists are the basis of a meal planning system designed by a committee of the American Diabetes Association and The American Dietetic Association. While designed primarily for people with diabetes and others who must follow special diets, the Exchange Lists are based on principles of good nutrition that apply to everyone. Copyright © 2003 by the American Diabetes Association and the American Dietetic Association.

"The Glycemic Index". American Diabetes Association. Copyright © 2003 by the American Diabetes Association and the American Dietetic Association.

"Calculate Your Body Mass Index". National Heart, Lung and Blood Institute (NHLBI), part of the National Institutes of Health and the U.S. Department of Health and Human Services. (2006) 1 p. On-line. Internet. September 2006. Available http://www.nhlbisupport.com/bmi

"Which of these are more motivating for you?" (© 1999-2006). 1 p. On-line. Internet. Available www.sparkpeople.com

"Movin"—Winter Burners: (2004). 2 pp. On-line. Internet. October 2006. Information courtesy of Ohio State University Medical Center. Available www.medicalcenter.osu.edu.

Zelman, Kathleen, MPH, RD/LD. "The Weekend Diet." Web MD Weight Loss Clinic. As seen on Web M.D. (April 6, 2006). 3 pp. On-line. Internet. July 2006. Available www.webmd.com.

"Get Moving, Stay Sharp". (February 2005). National Institutes of Health Info (NIH/OD). National Institute of Health Study. June 2005.

"IFATarget Heart Rate Chart". International Fitness Association. (1995-2004). 1 p. On-line. Internet. October 2006. Available www.ifafitness.com

"Taking a Heart Pulse (Heart Rate)". (1995-2006). 2pp. On-line. Internet. September 2006. As seen on Web M.D. Available www.webmd.com

Beets, Michael/Langrall, Rebecca. "Household Items, Serving Sizes". Wichita State University. (2006). 5 pp. On-line. Internet. September 2006. Available www.education.wichita.edu/caduceus

978-0-595-41465-9
0-595-41465-6

www.ingramcontent.com/pod-product-compliance
Lightning Source LLC
Chambersburg PA
CBHW030341290526
45785CB00004B/1561